Introduction to the Auditory System

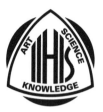

Edited by: Phyllis V. Wilson

Contributing Authors:
Patricia E. Connelly, Ph.D., CCCA
Jay B. McSpaden, PhD., CCCA, BC-HIS
J.C. Goldstein, MD, FACS, FRCSEd.
Kathy J. Harvey, CCC-A, BC-HIS
Alan L. Lowell, BC-HIS, ACA
William Schenk, BC-HIS, ACA

Published by:
International Institute
for Hearing Instruments Studies

Acknowledgements

This book is the third in a series of short volumes being published by the International Institute for Hearing Instruments Studies (IIHIS), the education division of the International Hearing Society.

Six distinguished authors, who are acknowledged experts in their field, took the time and energy to participate in this publishing project. Their contributions are immeasurable and the expertise they brought to this project is appreciated.

As editor of IIHIS textbooks, I would like to thank the authors for their contributions, also the International Hearing Society for their unwavering support of IIHIS.

Phyllis V. Wilson, Editor
IIHIS Administrative Director

Table of Contents

Chapter One

Anatomy and Physiology
of the Auditory System

Patricia E. Connelly, Ph.D., CCCA

Jay B. McSpaden, PhD., CCCA, BC-HIS

Anatomy and Physiology of the Auditory System

Introduction

Disorders of the auditory system can be understood only with a solid foundation in the physiology of a normal system. The focus of this text is to present the physiology of the auditory system as it relates to amplification and auditory rehabilitation issues. To that end, the objective of this text is to provide the foundations in anatomy and physiology that will allow the student to understand the connection between the acoustical event at the periphery and the perception of hearing involving the brain. In order to meet this objective, we'll review the anatomy of the outer ear and continue with that of the middle ear system. The cochlea will then be reviewed followed by the neural connections from the hair cells to the brain through the auditory nerve and central auditory pathways, including the temporal lobe and inter-hemispheric pathways.

Auditory physiology will begin where all acoustical hearing aid fittings begin, at the external auditory canal. Then, the middle ear's mechanical attributes and impedance matching functions will be presented, followed by cochlear physiology. Finally, the physiological substrates of the cortical event of "hearing" and binaural fusion will be presented. The functional target for every hearing aid fitting should be the preservation or restoration and maintenance of this "wired" system.

While proceeding with anatomy and physiology, it's essential that appropriate terminology be defined. Anatomical relationships are easier to conceptualize when using terms that establish location and/or spatial orientation. Proper pronunciation is essential to the presentation of a professional image. When these terms are presented in the text for the first time, they are *italicized*. Please refer to the Glossary at the end of the book for the definition and the pronunciation.

The External (outer) Ear

The outer ear is made up of the *auricle* or *pinna* and the external auditory *meatus* (EAM) or canal. The pinna is a skin covered flexible *cartilaginous* structure. Although the shape and contours of the ear vary from individual to individual, each has a number of common landmarks important to the hearing health clinician, and these can be seen in Figure 1.

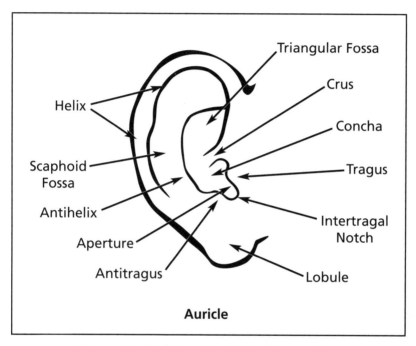

Auricle

Figure 1 – Landmarks of the External Ear

The outer edge of the pinna is called the helix. It is composed of skin covering cartilage. Directly posterior to the helix is the antihelix.

The lower part of the pinna is the lobule or earlobe. It contains no cartilage being made up of skin that covers *adipose* (fatty) tissue. The *tragus* is a triangular or pointed projection at the anterior opening of the external auditory meatus. Opposite this is the antitragus. Between them is the intertragal notch. The *concha* is a small cavity or bowl in the pinna that leads directly to the external auditory canal. These landmarks are important to know and recognize because they form a common terminology between the hearing health practitioner and the hearing aid industry, terms that convey considerable information for hearing aid shell and earmold fabrication.

The EAM courses *medially* from its *lateral* opening at the pinna to the tympanic membrane or eardrum. The opening is an irregular ovoid shape. It takes a tortuous course from lateral to medial with two bends and measures roughly 1.25 inches in length once fully matured at approximately age 12. A schematic is shown as Figure 2.

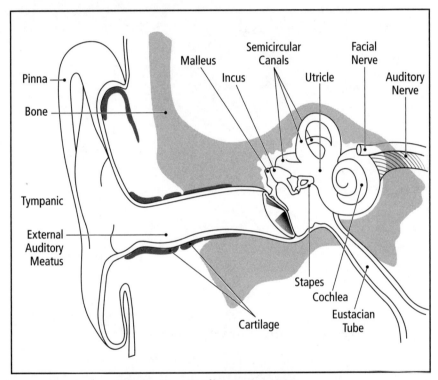

Figure 2 – Auditory Anatomy

The skin covering of the EAM is a continuous skin sac initiating from the growth center at the *umbo*. It is self-cleaning and transports dead skin, *cerumen*, and foreign material from the tympanic membrane to the opening at the pinna. The lateral one-third of the EAM is skin-covered cartilage with very little adipose tissue under the skin. It is in this outer one-third that the *sebaceous* glands and the *ceruminous* glands and hair *follicles* are located. There is a narrowing of the canal at the junction of the cartilaginous (lateral one-third) and *osseous* (inner two-thirds)

4

portions. This is called the ***isthmus***. The inner two-thirds of the EAM is comprised of skin that covers bone and both neural and ***vascular*** networks. There is no adipose tissue. There are pressure sensors located throughout the EAM, and the sensors located in the medial two-thirds are 2.5 times more sensitive than the more lateral ones.

The anterior wall of the external auditory meatus is directly adjacent to the posterior border of the ***mandible*** at the ***temporomandibular*** joint. In addition, the sensory route for the Xth (***vagus***) cranial nerve typically lies on the middle of the canal floor and up the posterior wall. The Xth cranial nerve has extensive connections with other brain structures involved with triggering nausea, mild chest pressure or a cough.

Tympanic Membrane

The tympanic membrane (TM) is roughly ovoid in shape corresponding to the shape of the EAM. It is attached to the temporal bone at the annular sulcus by the annular ligament. The TM is oriented not straight up and down, but rather obliquely with the inferior margin positioned more medially than the upper margin. The TM of the right ear points toward 1:00 and the TM of the left ear points toward 11:00. In other words, the top tilts toward the nose for each ear.

The TM is comprised of four layers. The lateral-most ***epithelial*** (dermal) layer is continuous with the skin that lines the EAM. The medial-most ***mucosal*** layer is continuous with the mucous membrane lining of the middle ear. Finally, there are two fibrous layers sandwiched between the epithelial and mucosal layers. Because of its translucency, structures located in the middle ear can be seen through the TM as shadows or fuzzy objects.

The TM is often referred to as the eardrum, however it is not flat like the surface of a drum. Rather, it is shaped like a cone with its point directed toward the middle ear. (see Figure 3). Because of this conical shape and its tilted vertical orientation, when a light is directed at it, a reflection of that light can be seen as a wedge or cone. It is known as the cone of light and is sometimes referred to as the TM's light reflex.

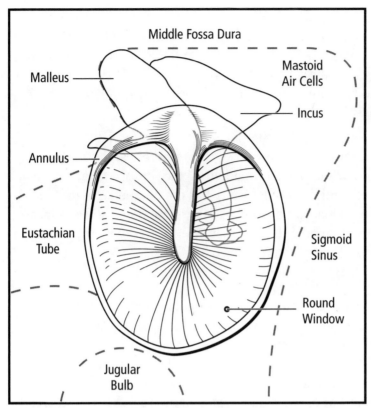

Figure 3 – Left Ear Tympanic Membrane Orientation

The TM is divided into two segments based on its elasticity. The superior portion is called the *pars flaccida* and is sometimes referred to as *Shrapnell's* membrane. It consists of only epithelial and mucosal layers. The *pars tensa* makes up most of the TM and has all four layers of tissue. The pars tensa is the energy efficient part of the TM in that it serves as the interface between the acoustic energy of sound waves and the mechanical system of the middle ear.

Structurally, the TM is divided into quadrants. The superior and inferior aspects are divided along the umbo. Anterior and posterior are divided along the length of the *malleus* through the umbo. The landmarks are conveniently identified by the quadrant through which they are typically visualized in the normal ear.

The color of the TM is pearly gray. It is highly *vascularized*. In the anterior-superior quadrant can be seen a small shadow that represents the *incus*, one of the *ossicles* (bones of hearing) located

6

in the middle ear space. The anterior-inferior quadrant contains the cone of light, the landmark of significant importance to the hearing health professional. It is used by all observers as an indicator of the health and functionality of the entire TM and middle ear system. The posterior-superior quadrant displays the long process of the incus and the *stapes* superstructure. Coursing through the middle ear space across both superior quadrants is the *chorda tympani* nerve. No landmarks can be typically visualized in the posterior-inferior quadrant.

There are two midline structures of importance. The umbo is the center of the TM where the *malleus* (another ossicle) attaches by way of a tiny ligament. The umbo appears as a small white or pearly dot at the TM's center (point of the cone). The second midline landmark is the *manubrium* (handle) of the malleus that can be seen extending from the superior portion of the TM inferiorly along the midline, stopping at the umbo. The attachment of the manubrium is only at the umbo and not continuously along its entire length.

Many landmarks are visible when the TM is viewed through the EAM and they are illustrated in Figure 4.

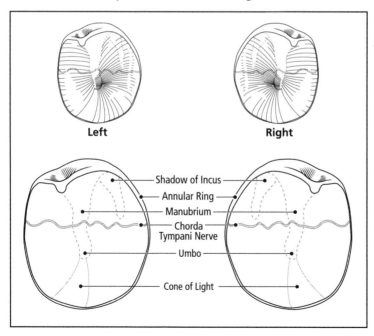

Figure 4 – Tympanic Membrane

Middle Ear

The middle ear is an irregularly shaped cavity that approximates a cube. Its walls are referred to by their anatomical orientations. The anterior wall separates the *carotid* artery from the middle ear cavity. The posterior wall is partially formed by the mastoid bone. The TM defines the lateral wall. The *cochlea* forms the medial wall. The roof of the middle ear space is also called the *tegmen tympani*. It is a very thin shelf of bone that separates the contents of the middle ear from the floor of the cranial cavity and base of the brain. The floor of the middle ear space separates the middle ear from the jugular vein. The contents of the middle ear space includes three bones, the tendons from two muscles, two nerves and several ligaments. Its interior dimensions are roughly the size of a small grape.

The middle ear ossicles are the smallest skeletal bones in the human body. They are commonly termed the hammer, anvil and stirrup because their shapes resemble those objects as seen in Figure 5. They are fully adult sized at birth and they do not grow.

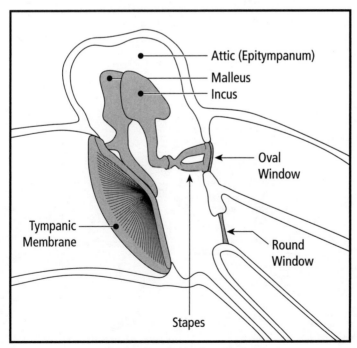

Figure 5 – Ossicular Chain

The lateral-most ossicle is the malleus or hammer, although it's really shaped more like a club. As previously stated, its manubrium attaches to the TM at the umbo. It is attached to and articulates with the body of the incus, the middle ossicle. The long process of the incus descends and turns at its terminus as the **lenticular process**. At this point the incus attaches to the head of the stapes by way of a tiny ligament. The stapes has a head, two **crura** (arms) and a footplate that fits into the oval window (**fenestra ovalis**) of the cochlea. The length of the stapes footplate averages approximately 1.5 mm. The stapes is oriented horizontally in the middle ear space. As a unit the ossicles are so small that they can be placed on the head of a penny and you can still see President Lincoln and read all of the words on the coin!

Ligaments independently suspended the ossicles in the middle ear space and attached each ossicle to one another. As a result of this independent suspension, any compression or expansion of the bones of the skull results in the application of inertia and subsequent movement of the ossicles relative to the skull.

The muscles of the middle ear are the **tensor tympani** and the **stapedius**. The tensor tympani attaches to the neck of the malleus by way of its ligament which arises from the anterior wall of the middle ear and courses posteriorly and superiorly to make the attachment. It is innervated by a branch of the Vth cranial (**trigeminal**) nerve. The stapedius tendon emerges from the posterior wall of the middle ear cavity to attach to the head of the stapes. Its neural supply comes from a branch of the VIIth cranial (facial) nerve. The stapedius muscle is the more clinically relevant middle ear muscle in that its contractions are measured for the acoustic reflex threshold and decay measurements made during immittance audiometry.

Two nerves cross the middle ear space. These are the VIIth (facial) cranial nerve and a branch of the Vth (trigeminal) cranial nerve called the chorda tympani. The facial nerve can lie across the stapes footplate, between the crura or on the **mucosa** of the medial wall of the middle ear space. The chorda tympani arises from the posterior wall of the middle ear cavity and can sometimes be visualized through the TM.

Another important structure associated with the middle ear is the *eustachian* tube (ET). Its opening into the middle ear is located on the anterior wall and it courses anteriorly from there toward the upper part of the *nasopharynx*. (back of the throat). The ET has a mucous membrane lining over muscles that run along its length. It is normally closed at its nasopharyngeal orifice, but this end opens and closes every third swallow in an adult.

Children's eustachian tubes are not as efficient as adults' in their open/close cycles. Additionally, the spatial orientation of the ET is grossly horizontal in children, thus impacting on the efficiency of its middle ear drainage function from gravity. As the head grows, the ET's orientation tilts until it approximates 45 degrees from horizontal in adults.

The Cochlea

The stapes footplate fits into the oval window of the *otic* capsule (cochlea). The otic capsule is simply another name for the *osseous* (bony) cochlea and balance system. These entities are not separable from the *petrous* portion of the temporal bone. Rather, they are an interconnected series of channels, tunnels and caves within that bone, which share common fluids and membranes and contain sensory receptors that are *innervated* by two functionally separate branches of a common nerve (VIIIth cranial nerve).

The osseous cochlea is coiled 2-3/4 turns from base to apex in a snail shape. Relative to other structures in the head, it is located directly medial to the helix of the pinna and directly posterior to the center of the eye. It is not oriented with its apex pointing straight up as is often conveniently portrayed in diagrams. Rather, the apex points forward and outward at an angle of 45 degrees from horizontal and from vertical as seen in the Figure 6. The uncoiled osseous cochlea measures approximately 31 millimeters from base to apex. It varies in width being wide at the base and narrow at the apex. It is fully adult formed at birth.

At this point it is important to introduce the two membranes important to cochlear integrity and physiology. The first membrane is located immediately medial to the stapes footplate and is called the membrane of the oval window. The second is the round window membrane. Its location is anterior to the oval window on the medial

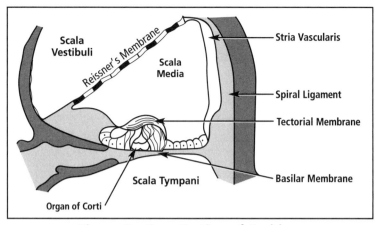

Figure 6 – Cross Section of Cochlea

wall of the middle ear. Specifically, it is located in the round window (*fenestra rotunda*) niche and is separated from the oval window by the *promontory*, the bulging of the *basal* turn of the cochlea into the middle ear cavity. These membranes serve to keep the cochlear fluids inside the cochlea.

Physiologically, the motions of the oval and round windows because of their locations at opposite ends of the fluid filled tube are reciprocal. The fluids of the inner ear are not compressible. In addition, there is no "air space". As a result, when the oval window moves inward, the round window moves outward.

The cochlea is divided into three compartments (or scalae) by two important ribbon-like membranes. These compartments are the *scala vestibuli*, the *scala media* and the *scala tympani*. The scala vestibuli is located just medial to the oval window membrane and stapes footplate. The scala media is wedged between the scala vestibuli and the scala tympani. Both the scala vestibuli and scala tympani are connected at the *helicotrema* located in the apex of the cochlea and they share a common fluid called *perilymph*. This fluid derives from cerebrospinal fluid and has a high potassium concentration and a low sodium concentration. The scala tympani terminates at the round window membrane. The scala vestibuli and scala tympani have no contents other than perilymph.

The scala media is also called the cochlear duct. It is separated from the scala vestibuli by **Reissner's** membrane and from the scala tympani by the **basilar** membrane. It is grossly wedge shaped as defined by the close proximity of attachment of these two membranes at the **modiolus** (central core of the osseous cochlea) and their divergent attachments at the outside edge of the cochlea. The scala media is filled with a fluid called **endolymph**. Like perilymph, it is derived from cerebrospinal fluid but is higher in sodium than potassium.

These endocochlear fluids are electrolytes. This means that they have ionic (organic, electrical) charge that differs from one side of the membrane to the other. In adults the differences average -80 millivolts. This voltage difference constitutes an organic and physiological battery.

On the outer margin of the scala media is the **stria vascularis**. This structure generates the electrical charge that drives the functions of the scala media. It provides nutrients, oxygenation and blood to the structures of hearing located within the scala media.

Contained within the scala media is the end organ or sensory receptor of hearing, the organ of **Corti**. It is made up of hair cells, supporting cells, a tunnel, a neural network and an overhanging membrane. These structures course continuously as a unit through the entire 2-3/4 turns of the cochlea from base to apex. These structures, that is, the organ of Corti, sit on top of the basilar membrane, which is attached on both sides to the inner and outer borders of the osseous cochlea.

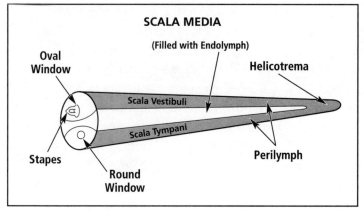

Figure 7 – Cochlear Fluids

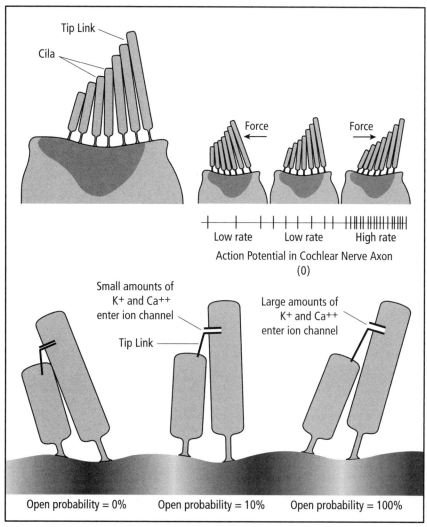

Figure 8 – Hair Cells

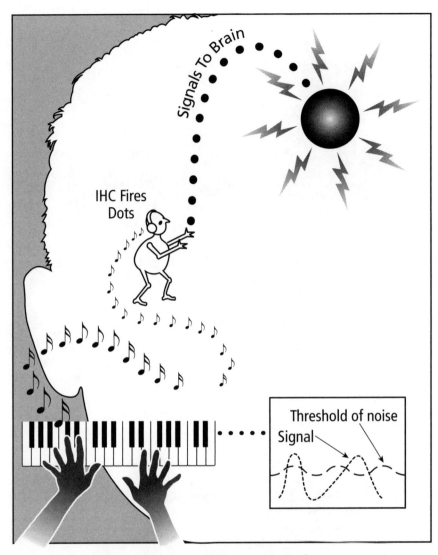

Figure 8B - Complete Model of the Ear

The organ of Corti has two types of hair cells that differ in shape and function. These are the inner hair cells (IHCs) and the outer hair cells (OHCs). There are one row of IHCs and three rows of OHCs. IHCs are shaped like a tulip, where as the OHCs are more cylindrical. The terms inner and outer stem from their locations relative to the modiolus, with the IHCs being closer to the cochlea's central core and the OHCs being located closer to the stria vascularis.

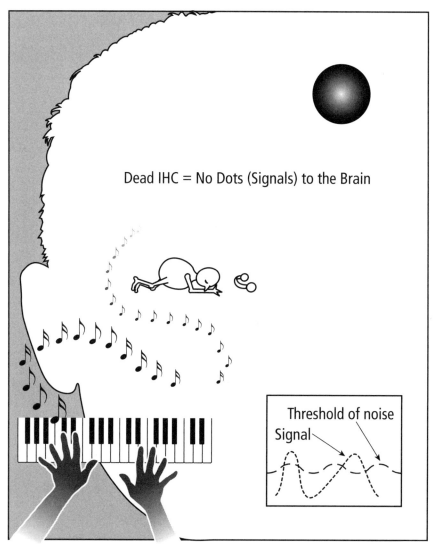

Figure 8C - Complete Model of the Impaired Ear

Both types of hair cells have **stereocilia** (hair like projections) on their free surface. The pattern of the stereocilia on the IHC is different than that of the OHCs. The stereocilia on the IHCs are arranged as a fan-like or crescent shape, whereas they form a W-pattern on the OHCs. The ends of the OHC stereocilia are imbedded in the inferior surface of the **tectorial** membrane. The stereocilia of the IHCs float freely in the endolymph.

The tectorial membrane is a gelatinous structure suspended over the top of the organ of Corti. It arises over the *spiral lamina* and is unattached at its outer edge. It extends over the top of the hair cells along the entire 2-3/4 turns of the cochlea. As a result of its attachments, movement of the tectorial membrane results in a pulling or shearing motion on the OHC stereocilia that stimulates those hair cells.

The IHCs and the OHCs arise from the basilar membrane at different angles that form an arch-like channel called the tunnel of Corti. This tunnel is filled with the endolymph of the scala media. It is simply a landmark of the organ of Corti.

The basilar membrane is attached on both sides along its 31 mm length throughout the 2-3/4 turns of the cochlear. It is widest at the apical turn of the cochlea and narrowest at the base. This may seem confusing given that the osseous cochlea itself is wider at the base than at the apex. This paradox is due to the basilar membrane's attachment by the spiral ligament to the modiolus. The spiral ligament is much longer at the cochlea's basal turn than at its apical turn.

The basilar membrane is made up of individual connected fibers that run transversely across the width of the membrane. These fibers are arranged side by side, one right up against the next. They are shorter, thinner and more taut at the basal turn, than those at the apical turn where they are longer, thicker and looser. As a result of this differential construction, the basilar membrane has a stiffness gradient that forms the foundation of the ear's ability to differentiate frequency.

The neurons that convey sound information to the central nervous system begin at the base of the hair cells. Of all neurons in the VIIIth cranial nerve, only 5% connect to the OHCs, whereas 95% are connected the IHCs. The OHC innervation is accomplished by extensive *arborization* (branching) of each neuron. In other words, one auditory neuron innervates or serves multiple OHCs. On the other hand, the IHCs have a one-to-one relationship with a single auditory neuron.

The auditory neurons from the outer hair cells course transversely through the tunnel of Corti toward the modiolus. Auditory neurons from both the IHCs and OHCs enter the modiolus where they begin to converge from all turns to exit the cochlea as a bundle. The cell bodies of these neurons aggregate in this central core to form what is known as the *spiral ganglia*. The neurons continue to course out of the cochlea exiting as a bundle called the auditory branch of the VIIIth cranial nerve. It is important to note that the nerve is arranged with fibers from the apical turn (low frequencies) coursing through the center of the bundle. The neurons from the basal turn (high frequencies) wrap around the circumference much like a coaxial cable.

The fibers of the VIIIth nerve are *myelinated*. This means that they have a physiological insulation that separates one from the other and facilitates the very rapid transmission of neural impulses from the organ of Corti to the central auditory nervous system. As a result of this *myelin* sheath, the neural impulses initiated at the organ of Corti arrive at auditory cortex of the temporal lobe in less than 10 milliseconds.

The Central Auditory System Pathway

Each auditory nerve courses medially through the internal auditory meatus of the temporal bone to the brainstem where it enters the central nervous system at the ponto-medullary junction, that is, the area of transition between the *medulla* and the *pons*. All auditory neurons from each ear *synapse* or relay at the cochlear nucleus on the same side of the brainstem. From the cochlear nucleus about 75% of these *afferent* (sensory) auditory neurons *decussate* or cross over to the other side of the brainstem through the trapezoid body. They then synapse at the *superior olivary complex* and ascend as a bundle or tract called the *lateral lemniscus*. There are additional synaptic junctions at the nucleus of the lateral lemniscus, at the *inferior colliculus* and at the *medial geniculate body* at the *rostral* pons / *caudal* midbrain. From the medial geniculate body, auditory fibers project or connect to the auditory cortex of the temporal lobe on the opposite side of the brain relative to the ear of origin.

It should be noted that auditory fibers cross over the midline at the nucleus of the lateral lemniscus and at the inferior colliculus in addition to the decussation at the trapezoid body. These multiple crossings result in the representation of each ear at the auditory cortex on both sides of the brain. This bilateral cortical representation of each ear optimizes the internal redundancy of the auditory system. As a result of these collateral pathways, an individual can sustain damage to the central auditory pathways and yet not demonstrate hearing loss. Of course, there might be auditory processing difficulties, but at least hearing loss would not impose a rehabilitative necessity.

Each synapse and decussation provides an opportunity for the auditory neurons to proliferate as the impulses proceed from the ear to the primary auditory *cortices*. For every one of the 30,000 fibers in the VIIIth cranial nerve, there is a geometric progression in the number of neural fibers from the periphery resulting in an estimated 10 million fibers from each ear at the auditory cortex. This proliferation further increases the redundancy of the human auditory system.

The cortical radiations from the medial geniculate body terminate the primary auditory cortex of the temporal lobe. There is a primary auditory area in each hemisphere of the brain. It straddles the top of the temporal lobe and wraps over around ***Heschl's gyrus*** into the ***Sylvian fissure***. The primary auditory association area surrounds that segment and facilitates the use of the meaning as identified in the primary area. It is also responsible for auditory memory and spatial acoustic cues.

Two broad bands of neural fibers course between and connect the brain's two hemispheres. The larger and primary band is a thick belt of fibers called the ***corpus callosum***. The smaller secondary band is at the same level of the brain but is located anterior to the corpus callosum and is called the anterior ***commissure***.

Once "meaning" has been assigned in the primary auditory cortex and auditory association areas of the temporal lobe, the fusion of signals into one coherent unit (perception) occurs as the signals are processed through these inter-hemispheric pathways, see Figure 9.

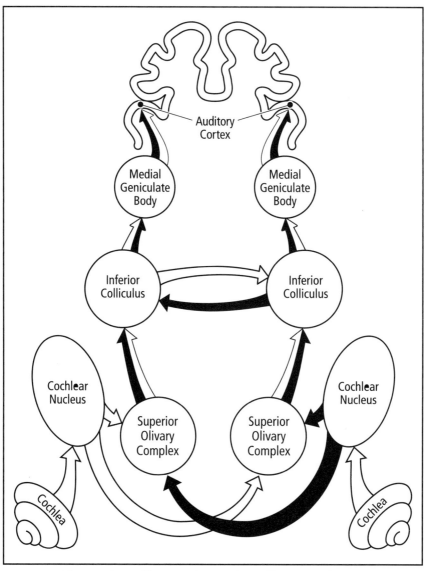

Figure 9 – Afferent Central Auditory Pathway

The Vestibular System

You need to keep in mind that the auditory system shares the temporal bone with the *vestibular* or balance system. The vestibular system is located posterior to the cochlea. Like the auditory system, it is comprised of tunnels and cavities hollowed out of bone that are occupied by fluid-filled membranous structures. These membranous structures house the sensory receptors that give us information about the position and movement of our bodies in space. This information is sent to the brain for processing by way of the vestibular branch of the VIIIth cranial nerve.

So, the VIIIth cranial nerve is actually made up of two separate branches; one conveys acoustical information to the brain and the other is responsible for information that influences our balance and sensations of body position and movement. Each neuron that makes up the VIIIth cranial nerve conveys only one type of sensory information. The VIIIth cranial nerve courses through the internal auditory meatus along with the facial nerve to enter the brainstem where the different branches diverge and travel to the various parts of the central nervous system in different pathways and tracts.

For additional information about the anatomy and physiology of the vestibular system, consult Martin, F: (Audiology, 7th Edition)

Auditory Physiology

The External Ear

The hairs and glands that line the EAM protect the ear canal and the TM, however they constitute the bane of the hearing health professional's daily practice. The oil and cerumen capture airborne particles and dust, which then combine with sloughed skin, *keratin* and other debris. This can accumulate and significantly impede hearing and/or hearing aid use. At the isthmus of the EAM, debris and/or cerumen can become lodged or packed in by the constant tamping action of earmold/hearing aid insertion or by cotton swabs. Overgrowth of EAM hair can become a problem if it impedes proper hygiene, impression taking and earmold/hearing aid insertion and retention. This is seen especially in elderly males.

The pressure sensitivity of the inner two-thirds of the EAM is increased by a factor of 2.5 relative to the more lateral area. This means that a hearing aid or earmold will be uncomfortable or painful if it causes more pressure than the ear canal can tolerate. Problems in the temperomandibular joint or any dental problems that alter the joint's normal alignment can also produce unacceptable pressures in a hearing aid or earmold fitting.

In addition, after an impression is taken, a small amount of blood can sometimes be seen in the EAM due to the vascular network just under the canal's thin skin. Pressure or stimulation in the canal can produce mild nausea, mild chest pressure and/or slight hoarseness during earmold or hearing instrument insertion and during the ear impression process due to the neural connections with the Xth cranial nerve. A reflexive cough (Arnold's reflex) can also result from such canal manipulation.

In terms of its physiology, the pinna collects sound waves and directs them into the EAM. In addition, the concha provides a *resonance* of approximately 10 dB at about 4700 Hz. The pinnae (plural of pinna) facilitate up-down localization. The EAM directs sound toward the TM and has a resonance peak at approximately 3500 Hz.

The combination of the pinna (notably the concha) and the EAM resonates at two peaks, one at about 2700 Hz and the other at about 5000 Hz. The amplitude of these resonances depends on the individual anatomy. This combined resonance influences high frequency hearing in that it naturally augments the amplitude of signals delivered with frequencies between about 2700 and 5000 Hz. It's easy to understand that the insertion of a hearing aid or earmold into the concha and/or EAM results in an elimination of these naturally occurring resonances that need to be restored through the hearing aid's frequency response.

The Middle Ear

This complex series of coupled membranes and bones acts as an impedance matcher. That is, the middle ear system acts to more efficiently transmit acoustical energy from the air to the cochlear fluid by matching the lower impedance of the air with the higher impedance of the inner ear fluid. It is a step-up transformer in that it builds up energy that will be lost when the mechanical energy interfaces with the cochlear fluids at the oval window.

The transformer action has two parts. The first is the ratio of the effective area of the TM to that of the oval window membrane. The ratio of the area of the pars tensa to that of the oval window is approximately 14:1. The second part is the mechanical advantage of the ossicular chain. This lever action of the ossicles introduces a mechanical advantage of 1.5:1. The combination of these ratios and the conversion of them into decibels result in a 27 dB increase in sound energy, as demonstrated in the formula:

N dB SPL = 20 log P1/P0, where, P1/P0 = Effective Areal Ratio times the Impedance Matching Transformer Action of the Middle Ear, or, 2 1/1.

The middle ear ossicular lever action exerts sound pressure from the TM against the stapes footplate in a piston-like action in and out of the oval window. The movement of the stapes at the oval window generates wave motion in the fluid or hydraulic system of the cochlea. Stapes footplate excursions replicate the frequency and amplitude (intensity) of the incident acoustical sound wave.

The increase in sound energy is needed to overcome the air-to-fluid impedance mismatch met by the acoustical signal. Without the middle ear impedance matching function, there would be a loss of energy from that acoustical signal at the cochlear fluids. The impedance matching function of the middle ear system mitigates the energy loss and makes the transfer of energy from the atmosphere to the inner ear much more efficient.

Another important function of the middle ear involves the *stapedius* and *tensor tympani* muscles. They both contract to increase the stiffness of the middle ear system and dampen its movement. The stapedius muscles contract when intense acoustic stimulation is presented to either ear. The contraction is consensual, that is, when one ear is stimulated, the stapedius muscle from each ear contracts due to their interconnections in the brainstem. It is this muscle reflex that is tested in the contralateral acoustic reflex threshold and reflex decay tests. It has been suggested that the contraction of these muscles helps to protect the inner ear from the damaging effects of loud, sudden sounds.

Energy Transduction

It can be said that the ear encodes the acoustic signal into a "language" that the brain decodes. This decoding by the brain is the perception of that acoustical event, in other words, the act of ascribing meaning to it.

Sound is that initial energy introduced into the ear, and it is in the form of acoustical energy. That energy interfaces with the TM where it is *transduced* into mechanical energy. The oval window membrane (just medial to the stapes footplate) is the interface of the mechanical system with the hydraulic system represented by the endocochlear fluids. The final transduction occurs at the base of the hair cell when the energy becomes electrochemical (neural). This is the only form of energy that the brain can process and/or decode.

Very simply, the following events take place when acoustical energy travels down the ear canal. First, the sound exerts positive and negative pressure against the TM where that acoustical energy is transduced into mechanical energy. Then, due to the step-up transformer action of the middle ear system, that is, the impedance matching function of the middle ear mechanism, this mechanical energy can overcome the energy loss at the air-fluid interface at the stapes footplate/oval window membrane. It is here that the parameters of the acoustic signal are now replicated as hydraulic events that we refer to as waves.

The geometry of the cochlea is such that irrespective of where the pressure is input to the system (that is, by air or by bone conduction), the wave always progresses from base to apex and back. The wave initiated at the oval window membrane travels along the 2-3/4 turns of the cochlea, passes unimpeded through the helicotrema and down the 2-3/4 turns of the scala tympani. Here its pressure is released at the round window back into the middle ear space. The osseous cochlea is completely fluid-filled and therefore, incompressible, so the endocochlear fluid does not move through this system, only the energy's wave-like motion passes through this system. This motion is transmitted to the basilar membrane causing wave-like motion in that membrane and all the structures resting upon it.

Now, for the initiation of the neural impulse. The organ of Corti is located on the basilar membrane which moves as influenced by the wave motion in the cochlear fluids. The stereocilia at the free margin of the hair cells are bent or sheared due to the inertial drag of the tectorial membrane. This shearing results in the transduction of this energy into the electrochemical event that initiates neuronal firing.

Theories of Hearing

The theories of hearing are physiologic statements about how we *think* this anatomic system works for both pitch perception and loudness coding. These theories are based largely on the transduction of middle ear mechanical energy into cochlear hydraulic energy. A single, precise explanation of how we hear remains unstated because so many aspects of auditory physiology remain unclear. More than one theory is needed to explain the behavior of the auditory system because it requires the synergy brought together by all of them. These hypotheses represent the integration of function of the different auditory structures. Truly, the whole is greater than the sum of the simple parts. These theories attempt to explain how the auditory system conditions the acoustic stimulus into a code that the brain can process.

Theories of hearing include those that assign pitch perception to the cochlea (Place Theories) and those that assign it to *retrocochlear* structures (Frequency Theories) It is actually a combination of these theories that provides us with a theoretical framework for how we hear.

The Place Theories explain pitch perception based on the inner ear performing a spectral analysis on the input signal, that is, the input is broken down into its individual frequency constituents. This spectral or Fourier analysis is made possible by the basilar membrane's structure that results in its differential sensitivity to signal frequency in that its basal turn responds best to high frequencies and its apical turn responds best to low frequencies. It can be thought of as being selectively "tuned" to each frequency at the different places along its length, thus the term "place" in Place Theory. So, a tone of 1000 Hertz (Hz) would best stimulate the segment or place on the basilar membrane that is tuned to 1000 Hz and the neural elements connected to this place convey the pitch information to the brain for processing.

The Traveling Wave Theory was proposed by von Bekesy to explain basilar membrane motion and its contribution to hearing. As previously mentioned, all acoustic signals introduced into the cochlea by way of the middle ear system travel as pressure waves initiated at the stapes footplate/oval window interface and travel apically from the base of the cochlea along the 2-3/4 turns in the scala vestibuli. The amplitude of the incoming wave reaches its maximum at the location along that 2-3/4 turns responsible for the encoding of that frequency. This location is determined by the basilar membrane's stiffness gradient that results from its unique structure.

The cochlea is a fluid-filled non-compressible system, so an energy release must occur; this happens at the membrane of the round window. When the energy is released through the round window membrane it is 180 degrees out of phase with the input initiated at the oval window membrane, thereby canceling the residual energy in the middle ear.

Research in auditory physiology has revealed that the Place Theory cannot account for all aspects of hearing. Frequency for place representation is known as tonotopicity. In reality, the nuclei of the brainstem auditory pathways and the primary auditory cortex are, in fact, tonotopically organized. It has been demonstrated experimentally that this frequency for place representations is maintained throughout the auditory system.

The Frequency Theory of hearing ascribes pitch perception to the firing patterns of the auditory neurons, rather than to cochlear elements as in the Place Theory. According to the Frequency Theory, auditory neurons fire at a rate equal to the frequency of the incoming signal. So, for a signal of 250 Hz, the neurons will fire at 250 times per second. This theory can only account for incoming signals up to about 400 Hz since experimental evidence indicates that the auditory neurons can fire only up to about 400 times per second. In 1949 Wever proposed the Volley Theory of hearing to account for the processing of frequencies higher than 400 Hz. He postulated that firings of sets of neurons are temporally interleaved to achieve cumulative firing rates well above 400 per second. However, it has been shown through experimentation that this theory can account for frequencies only up to about 4000 Hz, whereas the human auditory system is capable of hearing a range from 20 to 20,000 Hz.

So, considering these theories and their limitations, how do we hear? Hearing in terms of pitch perception is probably a combination of the Place (including the constructs about basilar membrane motion proposed by the Traveling Wave Theory) and Volley Theories. The Place Theory can account for high frequency hearing and the Volley Theory can explain low frequency pitch perception. Mid-frequency signals are probably heard through a physiological incorporation of the two.

How do these theories account for our perception of the other parameter of acoustic signal, amplitude? The Place Theories ascribe loudness perception to the amplitude of basilar membrane movement. Louder signals have greater amplitudes and these greater amplitudes cause the basilar membrane to move farther at its point of maximum displacement. This causes more impulses transmitted by the auditory neurons with a resultant perception of increased loudness. The Frequency Theory accounts for loudness perception based on a concomitant spread of motion across a larger area of the basilar membrane with higher amplitude signals, thus stimulating a greater number of neurons to fire at and near the frequency of the stimulus. More neurons firing convey more information to the brain with the resultant perception of a louder sound. Unfortunately, loudness perception is inadequately understood.

Of all of the sensory systems in primates, the auditory system is the most sensitive. Its exquisite sensitivity is one full order of magnitude (10 times) more sensitive than any other sensory system. As an example, if the eyes could see at the level that ears can hear, you would see bacteria. It is truly incredible that a system the size of the auditory system has such power. It can, in the healthy ear, resolve the "just noticeable differences" (referred to as the "JND's") for both frequency and intensity. It is Phenomenal.

This means that there is a specific row of cells, one IHC and three OHCs, that is uniquely responsible for the encoding of a given frequency. This place theory arrayed across the basilar membrane is the first of three *isomorphic* representations of this frequency specificity that are necessary for the generation, transmittal and decoding of a particular sound. Complex stimuli, such as speech and music, presented to the cochlea are broken down into their constituent frequencies in a kind of organic Fourier analysis, maintaining their relative amplitudes and keeping their correct temporal relationships, all of this information transmitted through the central auditory pathways. This signal conditioning into a code that the brain can process permits and facilitates the ultimate function of the auditory system, specifically, the assignment of meaning.

Before we leave the cochlea, it is necessary to discuss the most recent of the elegant theories of hearing. Proposed separately by Dallos and Kemp, it is referred to as the motor theory and was generated to explain the processing and transmittal of low intensity signals. This theory, the verification of which is now captured on video tape (Kemp), demonstrates that low amplitude signals initiate motion in the OHCs in such a way that they physically bend, move, elongate and tactilely stimulate the IHCs in the given location on the basilar membrane. The result of which is the perception of low intensity sound at that frequency.

A final parenthetic note: Previously, we referred to one of the three isomorphic representations as occurring along the basilar membrane. The other two place-differentiated structures are located in the ventral cochlear nucleus and the primary auditory area of the temporal lobe.

Hearing by Air Conduction vs Bone Conduction

When an auditory signal is introduced into the air and through it is captured by the ear in the manner described, it is an "air conducted signal". On the other hand, when that signal is introduced through the bones of the skull, and through the oval window membrane in sufficient strength as to set the entire mechanism into action, it is referred to as a "bone conducted signal". All signals, regardless of their point of origin, proceed from the oval window membrane to the apex.

Chapter Two

Hearing Disorders

J.C. Goldstein, MD

Kathy J. Harvey, CCC-A, BC-HIS

Hearing Disorders

The purpose of this text is to make the reader aware that when a person presents with a hearing loss there are many possible causes for this disorder. It is not sufficient to say that a person has nerve deafness, and that he needs a hearing aid. One must be careful to exclude a medical condition, treatable or not, as the cause of deafness. It is not our intent to make the reader an expert in all of these possible etiologies. Rather, the purpose is to make the reader aware of the possibilities and to discuss them briefly. The interested reader can go to the references and other medical literature for whatever depth and detail is desired.

The evaluation of the person presenting with a hearing loss begins with a detailed history of the present problem, associated symptoms (ear pain, discharge, tinnitus, dizziness), history of ear infections, trauma (both noise and physical), past medical history including ototoxic drugs and other diseases, eg. diabetes, cardiovascular, HIV. A detailed family history is important, inquiring about the parents, siblings, looking for possible genetic influences, pertinent physical exam, includes exam of the ear canals and visualization of the ear drums.

In taking the history and performing the physical exam, the reader should be aware of the "Red Flags" published by the AAO-HNS, any one of which, if present, is an indication for referral to a physician, preferably trained in treating diseases of the ear.

Red Flag Referral Rationale		
Symptoms	**Possible Related Factors**	**Complications of Delaying Treatment**
Pain in ear with normal tympanogram	Myofacial dysfunction syndrome, temporo-mandibular joint dysfunction, referred pain from tumor in the throat	Progression of disease or condition, may result in permanent disability or death
Pain, active drainage or bleeding from the ear	Otitis media, otitis externa, blocked pressure equalizing tube, cholesteatoma, perforation of the tympanic membrane, temporomandibular joint dysfunction	Temporary or permanent threshold shift, mastoiditis, facial nerve paralysis, meningitis, spread of condition to related or adjacent structures, osteomyelitis

Continued on next page

Red Flag Referral Rationale (continued)

Symptoms	Possible Related Factors	Complications of Delaying Treatment
Rapidly progressive or sudden onset hearing loss	Inner ear infection (bacterial or viral), autoimmune inner ear disease, acoustic neuroma, drug toxicity, perilymphatic fistula, Meniere's disease	Permanent hearing loss, deafness, facial paralysis, increase of symptoms requiring additional medical or surgical treatment
Dizziness	Bacterial or viral infection, Multiple Sclerosis, Meniere's disease, vestibular Or acoustic nerve tumor, epilepsy, Usher Syndrome, perilymphatic fistula	Increased risk of complications, including neurologic and cardio-vascular complications
Visible traumatic or congenital deformity of the ear	Genetic factors, accidental or deliberate trauma, atresia	Worsening of related conditions and/or symptoms, temporary or permanent hearing loss/ threshold shift
Conductive hearing loss or abnormal tympanogram	Outer or middle ear infection, foreign body or cerumen, eustachian tube dysfunction, otosclerosis or other ossicular involvement, cholesteatoma, atresia	Worsening of related conditions and/or symptoms, brain abscess, temporary or permanent hearing loss/threshold shift
Unilateral or asymmetric hearing loss	Acoustic neuroma, Meniere's disease, genetic factors, auto-immune inner ear disease, drug toxicity, acoustic trauma	Neurologic complications, facial paralysis, worsening of related conditions and/or symptoms
Tinnitus as a primary symptom	Acoustic neuroma, brain stem tumor, otosclerosis, Meniere's disease, neuro-vascular compression syndrome, myofacial dysfunction disease, Or other unknown causes	Need for extensive surgical or medical intervention, greater risk of complications from surgical or medical treatment, temporary or permanent hearing loss/threshold shift, hemorrhage, facial paralysis, multiple cranial nerve involvement

This is obviously a very abbreviated list of red flag referral factors. There are many great sources of information at your disposal. Investigate any of the above for more information. Increasing your knowledge will help in your ability to recognize potential problems and refer whenever it is in the patient's best interest.

Methods of hearing assessment are discussed elsewhere in this book. Suffice it to say, that hearing loss can be conductive, mixed, or sensorineural. Conductive loss is due to:

1. Blockage of the ear canal, congenital, wax, blood, or foreign body

2. Disruption of the tympanic membrane

3. Disorder of the ossicles in the middle ear

Otoscopy should reveal causes in 1 and 2. Ossicular disorders can be due to *disarticulation* caused by trauma or infection, or *stiffness* secondary to infection (adhesions) or diseases such as otosclerosis or Padgett's disease, or effusion. A tympanogram should indicate disarticulation, effusion, or stiffness. Any of these indicate referral to a physician is in order.

Sensorineural can be further defined as sensory (indicating pathology in the cochlea) or neural implying pathology medial to the cochlea. Sensorineural loss can be idiopathic or due to a variety of causes, including: autoimmune ear disease, diabetes, HIV, ototoxic drugs, multiple sclerosis, syphilis, polyarteritis nodosa, Cogan's syndrome, relapsing polychondritis, systemic lupus erythematosus, Wegener's granulomatosus, Sjogren's syndrome, Behcet's disease, and lyme disease. There is an adage that, any disease process that can adversely affect vascular and/or nerve tissue can play a prominent role in auditory function. Let us now review some of these possibilities in more detail.

1. Autoimmune Ear Disease (AIED)

Mention of this disorder brings to mind the name of Brian McCabe, MD, long standing chairman of Otolaryngology at the University of Iowa. Dr. McCabe introduced this entity in 1979 when he described a series of 18 patients that had this disorder. His sentinel case was a 25 year-old man with sudden loss in one ear, and progress loss in the other ear, as well as a unilateral facial paralysis. All of his symptoms improved when treated with decadron and cytoxan. McCabe describes AIED as typically bilateral, and in about one-third of patients associated with a unilateral facial paralysis. The diagnosis of AIED is made by the history, clinical findings, response to immune suppressive medications, and immunologic evaluation of the patient's serum. Patients who may have AIED include those with fluctuating unilateral or bilateral hearing loss with or without vestibular symptoms. There may be rapidly progressive or sudden deafness. Patients must be questioned about rashes, joint pain, visual or ocular symptoms. The mentioned disorders associated with AIED include Wagener's granulomatosis, polyarteritis nodosa (PAN), systemic Lupus erythematosus (SLE), Cogan's syndrome, relapsing polychondritis, Behcet's syndrome, and Sjogren's syndrome. Detail of these entities is beyond the scope of this chapter.

The laboratory workup includes an extensive array of blood tests looking for specific antibodies and other blood abnormalities. Clearly the responsibility belongs to the patient's physician. The interested reader can pursue the references for more detail.

2. HIV

Up to 33% of HIV infected patients have ear disease. Chandrasekar, Connelly et. al reported a study of 50 HIV positive patients and that sensorineural hearing loss is more severe in patients with more severe HIV infection. 34% reported aural fullness, 32% dizziness, 29% hearing loss, 26% tinnitus, 23% otalgia and 5% otorrhea. Certainly it is not common to take a sexual history and ask about illicit drug use in one appearing for hearing testing, but the reader should be aware that in the Chandrasekar study for risk factors for HIV infection, some 47% were infected through IV drug abuse, 12% through homosexual contact, and 67% through heterosexual contact. Multiple HIV factors were present in 25% of patients. Recall that the human immunodeficiency virus (HIV) is the cause of AIDS, the acquired immunodeficiency virus. The CDC, the Centers for Disease Control and Prevention, classifies HIV infected patients into three general categories: A, B, and C based on symptomatolgy with A being the earlier stage and C the most severe. These categories are further subdivided based on CD4, positive T lymphocyte counts. Temporal bone studies in these patients the gamut of pathological changes involving the middle ear, mastoid and inner ear from mild inflammatory through cholestatoma to cytomegalovirus and Kaposi' sarcoma of the eighth nerve.

Autometric results were not specific for this disorder, but rather varied as would be expected with otologic abnormalities present. In general, in the study cited, the automatic data showed worsening hearing loss with worsening HIV infection.

3. Diabetes

According to the CDC there has been an unexplained dramatic rise in the incidence of Diabetes in recent years. Some 7 million Americans have now been diagnosed with this disease. Some 20% of older Americans (over the age of 65) have Diabetes. Diabetes is the 6th cause of death in the US through such complications as heart disease, stroke, and kidney failure. Deafness is not as recognized a complication as blindness is; perhaps it represents a failure of the pancreas to produce insulin, the hormone which allows sugar (glucose) in the blood to be transported into cells to be used as "fuel." It also facilitates extra sugar to enter the liver for storage. In type II Diabetes the body makes insulin but in inadequate amounts. This is often associated with obesity and lack of exercise, and perhaps, since obesity is a recognized epidemic in this country, this may account for some of the increased incidence of this disease. Diet control and oral medications (hypoglycemic agents) may control the blood sugar levels. Otherwise, insulin injections may be necessary as they are in patients in type 1.

How can Diabetes affect hearing? Diabetes is known to cause small vessel disease, especially in the eyes, kidneys and extremities, and also nerve tissue damage as reflected in numbness and tingling in the hands and feet and cognitive defects by its effect on brain cells. Comment was made early regarding the importance of vascular and neural tissues in auditory function. We know that Diabetes causes small vessel changes in the eyes and kidneys; it is reasonable to suspect that this also occurs in the cochlea. Otoacoustic emissions testing reveals outer hair cell changes even when pure tone testing is normal. Evoked response testing in diabetics has shown that electrical signals may travel more slowly along the auditory nerve. These two facts indicate that diabetics may have more trouble understanding speech out of proportion to their pure tone impairment.

Great strides have been made recently in linking genetic mutations to disease. There may be as many mutations linked to hearing loss in humans, including one rare one linked to both hearing loss and Diabetes. The less than 2% of diabetics with this disorder have MIDD or Maternally Inherited Diabetes and Deafness. The hearing loss may precede the diagnosis of Diabetes. Men can inherit but cannot transmit this disorder. Only women can.

Perhaps the definitive study examining the association between Diabetes and hearing loss is now underway at the Portland, OR VA Medical Center. See the National Center for Rehabilitative Auditory Research at www.NCRAR.ORG for details.

4. Ototoxic Medications

It is well accepted that when one presents with a hearing loss, with or without vestibular symptoms, an inquiry must be made as to past exposure to topical and systemic medications. There are several classifications of ototoxic drugs:

A. **Nonantibiotic Ototoxic drugs:**

1. Chemotherapeutic

Cisplatinum causes a permanent high frequency in 62% of exposed patients. Vestibular symptoms are rare.

2. Loop Diuretics (furosemide, ethacrynic acid)

The ototoxicity seen here is caused by high doses causing edema of the stria vascularis, a transient condition that is reversible.

3. Salicylates

The ototoxicity here is demonstrated by a flat 10 to 20 dB flat loss seen in patients taking high doses and resolves in 24 to 72 hours after the drug is stopped. Tinnitus frequently precedes the hearing loss.

4. NSAIDS

The incidence of ototoxicity in the non-steroidal anti-inflammatory drugs is considerably rarer than with salicylates. However, when a SN loss occurs, it is permanent.

5. Quinine

This drug causes a high frequency loss that is reversible with short term use, but tends to be permanent with long term use. It often causes some vestibular symptoms.

B. **Systemic Antibiotic Ototoxicity:**

There are 2 classes of antibiotics capable of causing ototoxicity: the macrolides and the aminoglycosides.

1. Macrolides

Azithromycin, clarithromycin, erythromycin:

The first two drugs cause ototoxicity when given in large doses intravenously for serious diseases. This loss is probably irreversible. Erythromycin, on the other hand, can cause a loss after oral use. The incidence is low, the mechanism is not known, and it is likely to be reversible.

2. Aminoglycosides

Gentamycin, kanamycin, tobramycin:

The first aminoglycoside was streptomycin. Its ototoxicity and vestibulotoxicity was recognized early. Because of this the drug was modified early to dihydrostreptomycin as cochleotoxic as its predecessor was vestibulotoxic. The tree drugs named above are equally cochleotoxic. The incidence is low, probably 2 to 3% in one series, 8% in another. The ototoxicity is manifest first by tinnitus, and then by development of a high frequency hearing loss. The vestibular toxicity manifested by a gait disturbance, especially in the dark or when walking on a soft or uneven surface. The risk of toxicity is increased in patients with renal insufficiency or on some drugs (loop diuretics, chemotherapeutic agents). The cochlear pathology shows injury to the organ of Corti, especially in the basal turn. The outer hair cells are most susceptible. The vestibular pathology involves the christa ampullaris of the semicircular canals.

It is interesting that in our present medicolegal environment, the administering physician must practice defensive medicine and obtain peak and trough blood levels of the drug after each administration. Renal function must be monitored and an increasing serum creatinine is a warning sign of impending ototoxicity. With all of this, it is realized that there in no "safe" dose; ototoxicity is known to have occurred after a single dose!

There appears to be familial susceptibility, suggesting a genetic predisposition. Another good monitoring technique appears to be bedside measurements of the stapedial reflex and otoacoustic emissions, especially in the patient who develops tinnitus while on aminoglycoside therapy.

5. Noise

Noise induced hearing loss can be due to an episodic episode (an explosion, gunfire next to the ear) or due to chronic exposure to a level of 90 dB or more. OSHA standards allow decreasing times of exposure as noise levels increase in intensity. (see Table 1) According to Dr. David Lim, histopathologic findings on light microscopy of cochleae with noise induced hearing loss are similar to the changes seen in aminoglycoside induced cochleotoxicity: injury to the organ of Corti, always worse in the basal turn of the cochlea, and involving degeneration first of the outer hair cells, especially those in the inner row. Depending on the noise intensity and time of exposure the pathology can expand to involve other hair cells and even supporting cells.

Permissible Noise Exposures

Duration (Hours)		Sound Level Slow Response
32.0		80
27.9		81
24.3		82
21.1		83
18.4		84
16.0		as
13.9		86
12.1		87
10.6		88
9.2		89
8.0		90
7.0		91
6.2		92
5.3		93
4.6		94
4.0		95
3.5		96
3.0		97
2.6		98
2.3		99
2.0		100
1.7		101
1.5		102
1.4		103
1.3		104
1.0		105

Table 1

The reader should be aware of the concepts of temporary and permanent threshold shifts. The classic example is the steel worker in a noisy environment who goes to work on Monday with "good ears", but by Wednesday he is aware of an annoying tinnitus, and by Friday, he and his family are aware that his hearing is impaired, even to the degree of being socially inadequate. He spends Saturday and Sunday in a relatively quiet environment, the tinnitus disappears, the hearing improves, and Monday he returns to work. He had TTS, a temporary threshold shift. But with repeated unprotected exposure to what the Deafness Research Foundation has aptly termed "toxic noise" the TTS will become PTS, or permanent threshold shift, usually first affecting the 4000 to 8000 Hz frequencies, but then expanding to involving higher and lower frequencies if exposure continues. It is not known why some people's hearing is more sensitive to noise exposure than others, but such is the case. Another example of TTS, and reflective of the noisy environment in which we all live, can be demonstrated by leaving your car radio on when you come home one evening and letting it turn off when you turn off the ignition. The next morning when you start the car and the radio comes on at the volume setting you found comfortable the day before, it now is probably too loud! This reflects a TTS you had from environmental noise that abated with a quiet evening at home.

Our younger generations, reflecting the sense of invulnerability that youth has, is doing irreparable harm to their ears when they attend rock concerts without ear protection where the intensity of sound may approach the threshold of pain, 120 dB. There are ongoing multiple attempts to educate our young people to the danger of loud noise to hearing, and the need for hearing protectors by groups such as H.E.A.R. (Kathy Peck's Hearing Education and Awareness for Rockers) in San Francisco, but it is an uphill battle. Too many youths still feel the volume isn't loud enough until "you feel it in your bones". An audiologic study done years ago on college students revealed hearing levels in 20 year olds that the testers expected to see in 60 or 70 year olds. The resolution of this problem is multi -faceted including education, decreasing the noise outputs of machinery, both industrial and home (chain saws, lawnmowers, leaf blowers) and emphasizing the need to wear ear protection.

It must become fashionable to wear ear protectors at rock concerts! An exciting area of research today is the possible role of drugs such as antioxidants and magnesium in treating and/or preventing noise induced hearing loss.

6. Multiple Sclerosis

This is probably an autoimmune disease, perhaps instigated by a virus in genetically susceptible people, in which antibodies are developed which attack the myelin coating (the insulation) of neural tissues, resulting in disseminated patches of demylination in the brain and spinal cord. The symptoms and signs are extremely variable, depending on the number and sites of the lesions. The diagnosis is made by MRI showing the plaques. The reader should be aware that sensorineural hearing loss, with or without vertigo, may become a part of the disease or MAY BE a presenting symptom, just as a visual complaint may sometimes be. Age at onset is described as typically 20 to 40 years, affecting women more often than men.

If an otherwise healthy young adult presents with a sensori-neural hearing loss, with or without vertigo and without apparent cause, the possibility of MS must be considered, and so should referral to his/her physician.

7. Presbycusis

This is the term commonly used to describe the sensorineural hearing loss associated with aging when there is no other apparent cause. There has been much speculation as to possible etiologies. In a study of South Pacific natives where old people have hearing acuity we associate with our youth, is it because of their isolation from our life long noise exposure, or is it due to their unique lean diet? There have been attempts to associate the loss with elevated blood lipids, elevated cholesterol etc., but the search goes on. We know that men are affected more often and more severely than women. Stiffening of the basilar membrane and deterioration of the hair cells, stria vascularis, ganglion cells and cochlear nuclei may play a role in pathogenesis. Presbycusis appears to be related at least in part to noise exposure. The loss first affects the higher frequencies and gradually affects the lower, beginning to affect the 4 to 8 kHz range by 55 to

65, although age variation is considerable. The high frequency loss makes speech discrimination difficult, particularly when background noise is significant.

The on-going cutting edge of audiometric research is seeking to define these changes in the senior auditory system and relating the audiometric presentation to the specific pathology present. Central forms of presbycusis make speech processing especially difficult, and tests are evolving to define the extent of this. All of this will make the management of the growing numbers of our senior patients with hearing loss more effective.

8. Meniere's Disease

The classic patient with this disorder presents with quadruple symptoms: aural fullness, tinnitus, fluctuant sensorineural hearing loss and intermittant vertigo. These classic four symptoms are not present in all. The initial hearing loss is primarily low frequency but expands as the severity of the disease continues. The pathology is endolymphatic hydrops or too much fluid in the inner ear. One or both ears may be involved.

The initial treatment is medical: low salt diet, diuretics and symptomatic anti-vertiginous meds.

If medical treatment does not help, surgery may be considered. Endolympathic decompression or shunting of the inner ear fluid from the inner ear may be effective.

9. Acoustic Neuroma

Every hearing specialist must strive to not miss this tumor, if present. This is a histologically benign growth which has the potential to act malignantly by virtue of its location on the eighth nerve in the internal auditory meatus. One presentation may be poor discrimination in an ear with little or no pure tone loss.

The presence of this tumor must be ruled out in any unilateral sensorineural loss, especially with poor discrimination. This may or may not be associated with facial nerve impairment or vertigo, based on the size and location of the tumor.

The diagnosis may be made by MRI or CAT scan or other X-ray studies of the internal auditory canal.

SUMMARY

This chapter has attempted to review the medical causes of hearing loss, and clarify the instances when further medical evaluation and treatment is indicated. When the hearing evaluator feels it proper to refer the patient for further medical evaluation and/or treatment, the question sometimes arises as to which type of physician to direct them to. If he/she has an existing Otolaryngologist relationship, that would seem the referral to make with a detailed written evaluation of the problem and the reason(s) for referral with request for patient return for hearing aid fitting if it is agreed that this is appropriate. If the client does not have a relationship with an Otolaryngologist and the medical problem relates to the ear, then the evaluator should choose one he/she is comfortable with. If the problem is general medical, non-ear, then similar referral back to the client's primary care physician, again with a detailed written evaluation and reason for referral with request for return is appropriate. With the known increasing incidence of Otolaryngologists dispensing, there is sometimes a concern about losing the client if referral to such an Otolaryngologist is made. The ethical principals and position of the American Academy of Otolaryngology – Head and Neck Surgery is that in this situation the patient, after the ear problem is managed, should be returned to the referrer for fitting and further management. Hopefully these principles will be maintained and the good relationships between the hearing aid specialists and ENT's will long continue.

REFERENCES

"Antibiotic Ototoxicity: Pathophysiology, Management, and Medicolegal Implications". Spplmnt to ENT J. Jan. 2003

"Autoimmune Inner Ear Disease (AIED's): Autoimmune Diseases with Audio-Vestibular Involvement", www.audiologyonline.com/audiology/newroot/ceus/showclass.asp?id+103 4/8/2003

Chandrasekhar, S. S., Connelly, P., Brahambhatt, S. S., Shah, C. S., Kloser, P. C., Baredes, S., "Otologic and Audiologic Evaluation of Human Immunodefiency Virus-Infected Patients", American J. Oto. 21, Jan. Feb.: 2000

Chartrand, M. S., "Diabetes and Hearing Loss", www.Healthy hearing.com/healthyhearing/newroot/articles/arc_disp.asp?article_ id-27/24/2003

Cogan, D. G., "Syndrome of Non-syphlitic Interstitial Keratitis and Vestibuloauditory Symptoms". Arch Ophth,1945; 33:144-9

Gupta, R., Sataloff, R. T., Noise-Induced Autoimmune Sensorineural Hearing Loss", Ann ORL, 112: 2003

McCabe, B. F., "Autoimmune Sensorineural Hearing Loss". Ann. Otol, 88:585-589,1979

Mcdermott, D., and Vaughan, N., "Diabetes and Hearing Loss, Exploring Connections", Hearing Health, FALL, 2003

McDonald, T., DeRemee, R., "Wegener's Granulomotosis", Laryng. 1983; 93:220-31

Nageris, B., Ulanovski, D., Attias, J., "Magnesiium Treatment for Sudden Hearing Loss, Ann ORL, 113: 2004

"Presbycusis", The Merck Manual, 17thEd;1999: 681

Schwaber, M. K., Meyerhoff, W. L., Selesnick, S. H., Goldenberg, R. A.,"The Seven Warning Signs of Serious Ear Disease", Scientific Exhibit Presented at AAO-HNS Annual Meeting, San Diago, 1994

Chapter Three
Comprehensive Hearing Assessment

Alan L. Lowell, BC-HIS, ACA

William Schenk, BC-HIS, ACA

Comprehensive Hearing Assessment

Introduction

A comprehensive hearing assessment will be one of your most valuable tools in the measurement and evaluation of your patients' hearing potential. It will also help to determine a wide variety of hearing disorders and may provide valuable information as to where or what is causing or contributing to a disorder.

A basic hearing assessment includes pure tone air and bone conduction audiometry and a battery of speech tests that include Speech Reception Threshold (SRT), Most Comfortable Listening Level (MCL), Uncomfortable Listening Level (UCL) and Speech Discrimination also known as Word Recognition (WR) test. An increasing number of hearing healthcare professionals are including tympanometry and acoustic reflex as part of customary test protocols. The individual and collective results of these tests reveals the site(s) and cause(s) of the more common hearing disorders routinely facing hearing healthcare professionals. Moreover, evaluation of the test results will serve as the basis for selecting the most appropriate amplification system. It also helps clinicians determine the need for referral to another professional.

A case history and inspection of the ear canal and eardrum (otoscopy) is an integral part of a comprehensive hearing assessment and most often is taken prior to any testing. However, the depth of a patient's case history generally is determined by the purpose for conducting the evaluation in the first place. A case history will often include information about a patients' medical, family, hearing and communication history as well as life style, preferences and needs assessment.

More recent tests such as loudness growth and discrete UCL measurements, tests that determine various levels of loudness and comfort will be discussed at the end of this text. Masking, Otoimmitance measures that include tympanometry and acoustic reflex and tuning fork tests will also be discussed.

Audiometry

Sounds are normally conducted to and through the outer ear by small changes in air pressure known as acoustic energy (air conduction). Air conducted signals provide the best transmission for human hearing. Audiometry helps to detect a hearing disorder(s), the degree of hearing loss, if any, and provides information that will help to locate the site(s) within the hearing mechanism that may be affected.

In order to measure hearing, a threshold of hearing must be established. This is accomplished by presenting the test ear with both pure tone and speech signals. To establish a threshold, the lowest intensity level an individual can either hear a pure tone, or in the case of speech, repeat words correctly fifty-percent of the time, must be obtained. A comparison between air-conducted signals (pure tone) and bone-conducted signals (through the mastoid process of the temporal bone) will help to determine the nature, location and cause of a hearing disorder. It will help to determine if a disorder is conductive, sensorineural, mixed or is categorized central deafness.

Adults who typically visit a dispensing practice are more likely to experience a sensorineural disorder and far less likely to be affected by a retro-cochlear disorder (involvement beyond the cochlea). A retro-cochlea disorder may involve the cochleo-vestibular nerve (VIII Cranial), brainstem or cortex. Any of these may cause or contribute to hearing loss.

Audiometric Equipment

In order to conduct an accurate comprehensive hearing assessment the following minimum equipment must be used and test conditions must be met:

1. Pure tone audiometer with both air and bone conduction capability and masking, calibrated per ANSI S3.6 1996

2. Telephonic Dynamic Headset (TDH) or insert earphones

3. Bone Oscillator

4. Speech audiometer or Master Hearing Aid (PMI) calibrated per ANSI S3.6 1996

5. Test environment that does not exceed ambient noise levels that can interfere with the accuracy of the test

6. Seating arrangement that prevents your patient from seeing your motions, gestures or reading your lips

7. Clearly understood and followed instructions

8. A testing technique that does not establish a presentation pattern that may cause a reflex response

The Audiometer

A clinicians' most useful and valuable piece of equipment is the audiometer. It provides physical measurements of sound as they relate to intensity (loudness) and frequency (pitch). The audiometer is the most appropriate piece of equipment that measures hearing sensitivities. Throughout recent time audiometric equipment has been calibrated to a specific standard that ensured accurate and properly interpreted measurements. Among the various standards implemented over the years are the International Standards Organization (ISO) and American Standards Association (ASA). Since 1977 audiometers have been calibrated in accordance with the American National Standards Institute (ANSI) and currently must be in compliance and calibrated to ANSI standard S.3.6 1996.

Figure 1 lists the key components of an audiometer and a brief description of their use and purpose.

The standard components of a comprehensive hearing evaluation are routinely conducted as follows, although not required in any specified order:

- Weber   tuning fork test
- Rinne'   tuning fork test
- Pure tone / air conduction   threshold test
- Pure tone / bone conduction   threshold test
- Most Comfortable Listening Level   (MCL)   suprathreshold
- Speech Reception Threshold   (SRT)   threshold test
- Uncomfortable Listening Level   (UCL)   suprathreshold
- Speech Discrimination   (PB Max 50)   suprathreshold

HEARING EVALUATOR

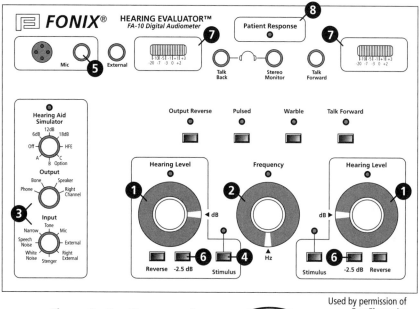

Figure 1 - Key Components

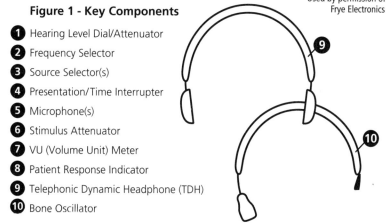

1. Hearing Level Dial/Attenuator
2. Frequency Selector
3. Source Selector(s)
4. Presentation/Time Interrupter
5. Microphone(s)
6. Stimulus Attenuator
7. VU (Volume Unit) Meter
8. Patient Response Indicator
9. Telephonic Dynamic Headphone (TDH)
10. Bone Oscillator

Used by permission of
Frye Electronics

Figure 1

Establishing a Threshold

Hearing measurements are made utilizing the decibel (dB) and establishing various intensity levels. Several methods are routinely utilized to establish a threshold of hearing. Unless contra-indicated, thresholds should be established on the better ear first. A hearing threshold is obtained by determining the lowest hearing level at which that patient can just hear a test tone or repeat a word correctly 50% of the time. The most common method is known as the descending/ascending method. This method requires that a signal (pure tone, speech, etc.) initially be presented at intensity levels easily heard by the patient. A signal is presented several times at that intensity level to ensure it is heard and/or understood. The signal is reintroduced several times at each level decreasing the presentation level in 10 dB increments until it is no longer heard (for pure tone audiometry) or repeated correctly (for speech audiometry). The signal is reintroduced increasing the presentation level in 5 dB increments until it is heard or repeated correctly at least fifty percent (50%) of the time. While other methods to determine thresholds are perfectly acceptable, the descending/ascending method is strongly recommended as it permits a signal to be easily identified by the listener and helps to avoid hearing fatigue. Both pure tones and speech reception thresholds (SRT) may be obtained through use of the descending/ascending method, see Figure 2.

Diagram of Descending/Ascending Method

For example: Frequency is 1000 Hz. Right Ear.
Present tone at:

40 dB	Tone is heard	Descending Technique
30 dB	Tone is heard	(Down 10 dB)
20 dB	Tone is heard *	
10 dB	No response.	
15 dB	No response.	Ascending Technique
20 dB	Tone is heard *	(Up 10 dB)
10 dB	No response.	Bracketing No. 1
15 dB	No response.	(Down 10 dB, up 5 dB steps until heard)
20 dB	Tone is heard *	
10 dB	No response.	Bracketing No. 2
15 dB	No response.	(same as No. 1)
20 dB	Tone is heard *	

The recorded threshold is 20dB at 1000Hz
* If the response is "yes", drop down 10dB.
  If no response, increase 5dB

Figure 2

Test Frequencies

Pure tone measurements are obtained by establishing thresholds at each octave between 125 Hz – 8000 Hz. Thresholds at the half octaves must be established anytime the thresholds between octaves shift 20 dB or more. However, it is becoming highly acceptable to routinely test the half octaves especially at 3000 Hz. A loss at the frequency will often strengthen both a patient's motivation and acceptance for amplification. The chart below illustrates two acceptable test progressions used in pure tone audiometry:

Carhart Method	Classic Method
1000 Hz	1000 Hz
500 Hz	2000 Hz
250 Hz	**3000 Hz**
125 Hz	4000 Hz
2000 Hz	8000 Hz
3000 Hz	500 Hz
4000 Hz	250 Hz
8000 Hz	125 Hz

Pure Tone Air Conduction

Equipment: Calibrated pure tone audiometer and TDH headsets or insert earphones.

Figure 3 illustrates a blank audiogram onto which audiometric results are recorded. Every audiogram should include an audiogram key describing what each symbol represents so that any healthcare professional would know how to correctly interpret the results. However, a red **O** for the right ear and blue **X** for the left ear are used universally for pure tone air conducted thresholds.

The frequencies (pitch) listed across the top and bottom of the audiogram represent the frequencies where thresholds are obtained. Typically, the audiogram will include frequencies listed from 125 Hz (low pitch) – 8000 Hz (high pitch). However, most speech signals fall between 500 Hz – 4000 Hz. The intensity levels measured in decibels (dB) are listed vertically on both sides of

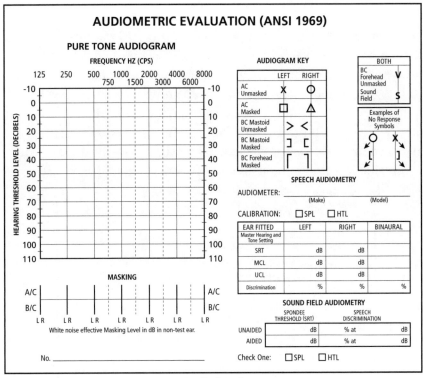

Figure 3 - Blank Audiogram

the audiogram. Thresholds are recorded from -10 dB representing perfectly normal hearing to 110 dB which represents a profound hearing loss (deafness). The further down the audiogram thresholds are recorded the more severe the hearing loss. Figures 4 - 7 illustrate various degrees of hearing loss. A pure tone average (PTA), often used to describe the severity of hearing loss is an arithmetic average of thresholds at 500 Hz, 1000 Hz & 2000 Hz. However, when thresholds between these octaves decline more than 15 dB a PTA is obtained by averaging the two frequencies closest to normal hearing as in figure 5. Besides interpreting the severity of a hearing loss close consideration is also given to its configuration such as flat, gradual, precipitous, fragmented, reversed, etc. Figures 8 - 12 illustrate various types of loss configurations.

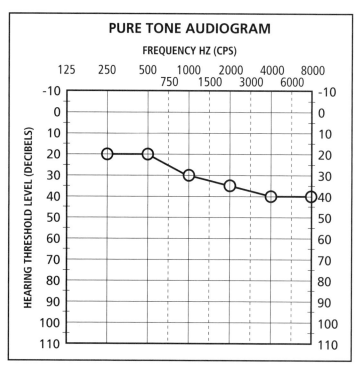

Figure 4 - Mild Loss

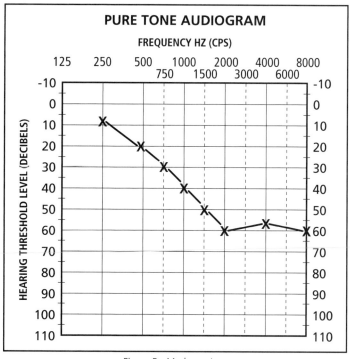

Figure 5 - Moderate Loss

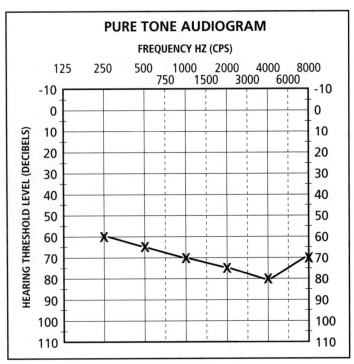

Figure 6 - Severe Loss

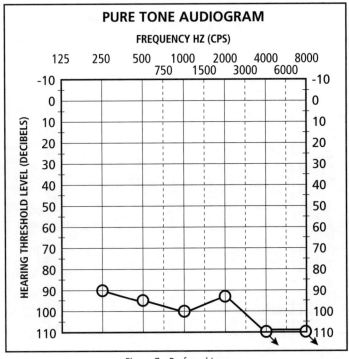

Figure 7 - Profound Loss

54

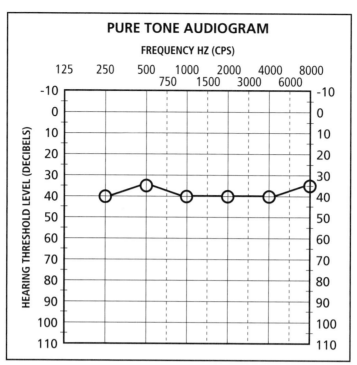

Figure 8 - Flat Loss

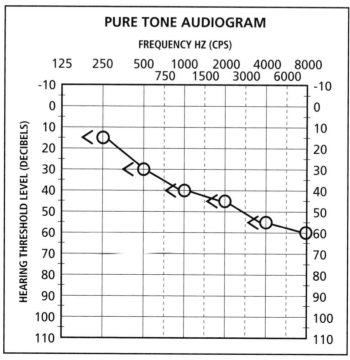

Figure 9 - Gradual Loss

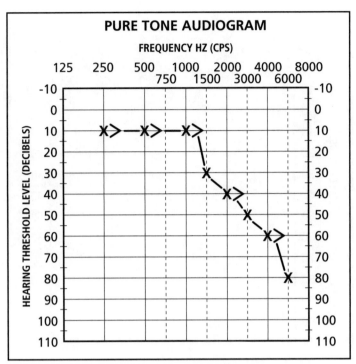
Figure 10 - Precipitous Loss

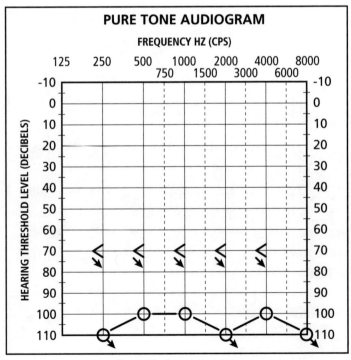
Figure 11 - Fragmentary Loss

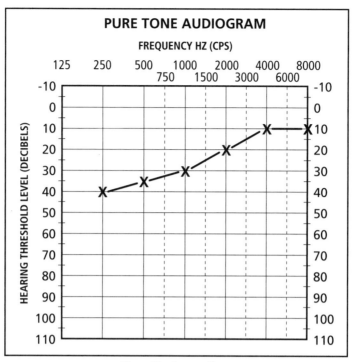

Figure 12 - Reverse Slope

Pure Tone Bone Conduction

Equipment: Pure tone audiometer; bone oscillator; TDH headset or insert earphones (for masking)

Unlike pure tone air conduction scores, bone conduction thresholds *only* measure the sensitivity of the cochlea. By placing the bone oscillator on the most sensitive (responsive) area of the mastoid process of the temporal bone, the test tones by-pass the outer and middle parts of the ear. If bone conduction thresholds are similar to those of air conduction then the hearing loss, if any, is sensorineural (figure 13). On the other hand, if the difference between the air and bone conducted scores are greater than 15 dB then the hearing loss is conductive or mixed (figures 14 and 15). A pure conductive hearing loss only involves an obstruction or breakdown in either the outer or middle parts of the ear or both.

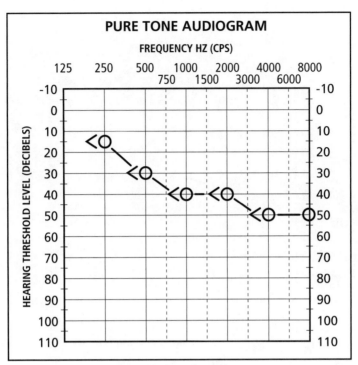

Figure 13 - Sensorineural Loss

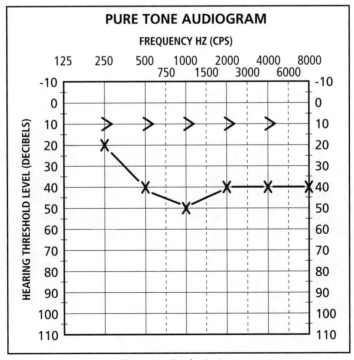

Figure 14 - Conductive Loss

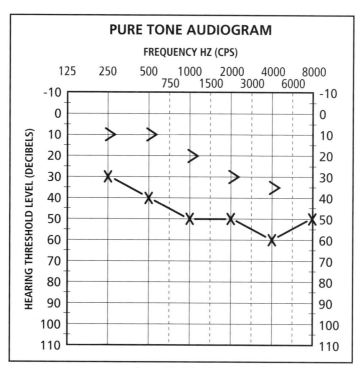

Figure 15 - Mixed Loss

A mixed hearing loss has both a sensorineural and conductive component (figure 15). In other words part of the loss is due to a disorder of the cochlea (sensorineural) and part is due to an obstruction or breakdown in the outer or middle ear (conductive).

As in pure tone conduction, bone conduction thresholds are obtained utilizing the same methods with one exception. The limits of intensity level (decibels) and test frequencies are determined by the limits of the test equipment. For example, in most cases 70 dB is the loudest level and 4000 Hz is the highest frequency that can be accurately measured. Unmasked bone conduction symbols are recorded with a < for the right ear and a > for the left ear. Bone conduction scores obtained with masking are indicated with a [for the right ear and a] for the left ear. We will be discussing masking later in this text.

Speech Audiometry

Equipment: Speech audiometer or master hearing aid (PMI); TDH headset or insert earphone.

As you assess hearing, you will find that people with almost identical pure tone audiograms often show wide differences in speech scores. As in pure tone audiometry, speech audiometry not only establishes a threshold for speech reception known as the speech reception threshold (SRT), it also establishes various comfort and uncomfortable listening levels and discrimination scores. A comparison of pure tone and speech results often will help determine whether you should proceed with a hearing aid fitting or refer your patient to another professional. It also is a key element in the selection process or in deciding that amplification will be of no assistance. In addition to the SRT, three other tests all considered part of a comprehensive audiometric hearing assessment are administered. These tests are the MCL, UCL and Word Recognition (WR) tests. First, let us discuss the various types of testing equipment.

Speech Audiometer Vs Master Hearing Aid

Understanding the difference between a speech audiometer and master hearing aid, also known as a Pressure Measuring Instrument (PMI) requires that zero decibel always have a reference and knowing the difference between measurements made in HL (hearing level) and SPL (sound pressure level). For example, both air and bone conduction audiometry measurements are always recorded in HL. On the other hand, speech testing can be measured in either HL or SPL depending upon the type of equipment used. Measurements obtained using a speech audiometer are made in HL. Let us explore the differences further.

Figure 16 illustrates an audiometric zero curve line that shows a greater amount of sound pressure is needed in the lower frequencies to make them sound equally loud as the higher frequencies. Pure tone audiometers are calibrated in HL with an average of ten decibels (10 dB) of sound pressure built into audiometric zero. This is why most audiograms include a space for – 10 dB threshold measurements (Figure 17). Patients with perfect hearing may hear at -10 dB. Speech audiometers are also calibrated in HL, however, when placed into speech mode an average of twenty decibels (20 dB) of sound pressure is built into speech audiometric zero. So, measurements made in HL either have an average of 10 dB built into audiometric zero for pure tone audiometry or 20 dB for speech.

However, hearing aids are measured in Sound Pressure Level (SPL) where zero dB is equal to .0002 dyne/sm which is the weakest sound that the best human ear is able to hear. Speech results can be established by use of a speech audiometer or a master hearing aid. Master hearing aids function similar to speech audiometers, however, they are calibrated in SPL and have the ability to more closely simulate how hearing aid(s) would sound. This information is particularly useful when selecting hearing aids most appropriate performance characteristics and specifications. Depending upon the type of speech equipment used to obtain your results, a conversion formula from HL to SPL may need to be applied.

Audiometric Zero

Frequency	dB SPL (Through TDH-39 headphones)	dB SPL Through TDH-49 & 50 headphones)
125Hz	45.0dB	47.0dB
250Hz	25.5dB	26.5dB
500Hz	11.5dB	13.5dB
750Hz	8.0dB	8.5dB
1.K	7.0dB	8.5dB
1.5K	6.5dB	7.5dB
2.K	9.0dB	11.0dB
3.K	10.0dB	9.5dB
4.K	9.5dB	10.5dB
6.K	15.5dB	13.5dB
8.K	13.0dB	13.0dB

Figure 16 - Audiometric Zero

HL to SPL Conversion

(To HL level add or subtract to find SPL)

Frequency

250Hz	add	15dB
500Hz	add	9dB
1.K	add	3dB
2.K	subtract	3dB
4.K	subtract	4dB
8.K	add	13dB

A 250 Hz sound needs to be 15dB SPL before a normal hearing person is just aware of it, whereas it only takes 3dB SPL for 1000Hz sound to become audible.

Figure 17 - HL to SPL Conversion

Most Comfortable Listening Level (MCL)

The purpose of the MCL is to establish a most desirable and comfortable listening level for conversational speech. This measurement provides valuable information in the selection of an appropriate hearing aid circuit. The MCL may be established by using various methods that include recorded speech or unemotional live voice (no inflection). Most often an MCL will be established at or between 20 dB - 30 dB above the SRT. The MCL often should precede any other test as it permits your patient to receive instructions or have a conversation without having to strain to hear. It's important to note when establishing the MCL, as with all other speech tests, the signals should be presented at calibrated levels. The test equipment must be closely and continually monitored to ensure that it remains in speech calibration throughout the test. This is accomplished by monitoring the vu (volume units) meter. It is used to calibrate the test materials such as tape, CD or live voice signals.

Speech Reception Threshold (SRT)

The purpose of the SRT is to establish a threshold whereby speech is initially heard and understood. The SRT should not be confused with the SAT (*Speech Awareness Threshold*) or SDT (*Speech Detection Threshold*). The SRT provides valuable information as it relates to the confirmation of pure tone test scores. Generally, in cases of a gradual sensory presbycusis hearing loss, the SRT will fall within 10 dB of the pure tone average (PTA). On the other hand, an SRT greater than 10 dB of PTA along with other indicators may point to a *retro-cochlea disorder* (beyond the inner ear) that may require medical referral.

As in other threshold testing the SRT is established using the descending/ascending method. Spondaic words, two syllable words with equal stress placed on both syllables, such as inkwell, armchair and baseball are presented in groupings of three, descending in 10 dB steps until they are no longer heard correctly. The words are increased in 5 dB increments until at least 50% of the words are repeated correctly. The SRT is also used to establish the *dynamic range* (DR) by subtracting it from the Uncomfortable Listening Level (UCL). The dynamic range identifies the parameters and useful range in which a hearing instrument will operate most effectively. The dynamic range is also known as the *auditory area*.

Uncomfortable Listening Level (UCL)

The UCL is one of several names given to a test that establishes an intensity level where sounds (usually speech signals) are most uncomfortable (below the threshold of pain). Names for similar tests include *Threshold of Discomfort* (TD) and *Loudness Discomfort Level* (LDL). Other tests, that use pure tone signals such as *Discrete UCL* and *Loudness Growth Measurements* will be discussed later. A wide variety of speech signal(s) and test methods may be used to establish the UCL. To establish a UCL the intensity level control is increased from the MCL in 5 dB increments until the signal presented is very uncomfortable but below the threshold of pain. It is a vitally important measurement as it determines the maximum output level a patient can tolerate with a hearing instrument(s). Its worth noting that the majority of today's hearing instruments have some form of *automatic signal processing* (ASP) capability and therefore are less likely to saturate and exceed a patients' threshold of discomfort.

Word Recognition (WR) Test

Unlike other audiometric tests, word recognition is scored in percentages based on words repeated correctly when presented at the MCL. In other words, how improved would ones ability to understand speech be by wearing hearing aids. *Word recognition* is one of four key elements necessary for a patient to obtain the greatest satisfaction level from hearing aids. The other elements are physical comfort, sound quality and aesthetics.

Word recognition tests may also be referred to as the PB Max. These are phonetically balanced monosyllabic words (single syllable) such as twins, owl, ace and low, that are presented at MCL from a list of 50 words also known as PB Max 50. A variety of lists are available, most of which are similar and accomplish the same results. A minimum of 25 words from the same list must be presented monaurally and scored in percentages for words repeated correctly. For example, 20 words repeated correctly from 25 words presented = 80%. Binaural word recognition testing should follow, as it will indicate what improvement if any, may be derived from wearing hearing aids in both ears. When obtaining binaural word recognition scores it may be necessary to reduce the presentation levels by 5 dB to offset a *central effect*. There are instances when wearing hearing aids in both ears may produce poorer aided speech discrimination scores. This is known as *binaural degradation*, in which case a monaural fitting should be strongly considered.

Another method to establish speech discrimination scores is through the use of the modified rhyme word test. The *modified rhyme* test is given to a patient who reads the words as they are presented at MCL and is instructed to circle the word that is heard. The words are listed in 25 groupings of three as seen below. They are not

1. Rat	2. Teach	3. Kit
Cat	Reach	Fit
Bat	Peach	Sit

necessarily phonetically balanced but have reasonable phonemic similarity. Clinicians, who themselves have hearing loss, may prefer this method of testing to ensure that the test is scored correctly.

Masking

A masking noise is introduced to a non-test ear so that it cannot respond to or hear a signal simultaneously being presented to a test ear. Establishing an effective amount of masking so that the ears are not either over or under-masked requires a thorough understanding of masking concepts too vast to cover in this text. However, for pure tone air conduction audiometry, masking must be introduced to the non-test ear in those frequencies where air conducted thresholds in the test ear exceed bone conduction thresholds in the non test ear by 40 dB or greater as seen in Figure 18.

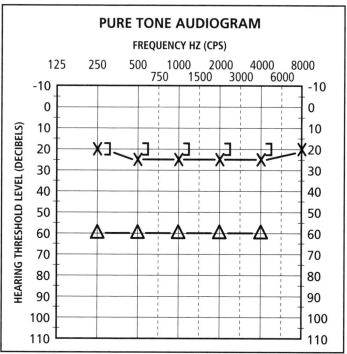

Figure 18 - Monaural Masking

Since bone conduction signals are introduced through the mastoid process of the temporal bone it's possible that even if the hearing in both ears is symmetrical the non-test ear may respond to and hear the tone presented to the test ear. Therefore, while it is acceptable and in fact good practice to always mask the non-test ear for bone conduction, it must be masked when it exhibits an air/bone gap as seen in Figure 19. Generally, if masking was necessary for pure tone air conduction it must also be used when obtaining speech scores.

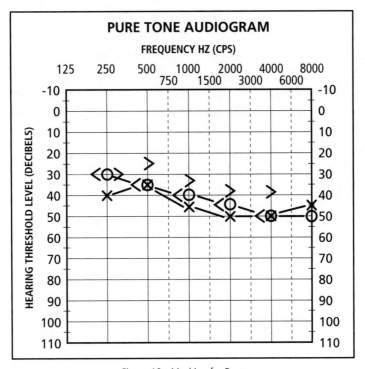

Figure 19 - Masking for Bone

Discrete UCL

Earlier, we briefly discussed that the dynamic range was determined by subtracting the SRT from the UCL and that this was the area (auditory area) that a hearing aid would perform most effectively within. Instead of using speech signals, discrete UCL's are determined by presenting pure tones at each discrete frequency between 125 Hz – 8000 Hz. Like speech signals, the intensity levels are increased in 5 dB steps until they are heard just below the threshold of pain. This often is a more desirable method especially when considering advanced circuitry such as automatic signal processing (ASP). Many ASP circuits can be programmed not to exceed the UCL at different frequencies. Figure 20 illustrates an audiogram with discrete UCL's.

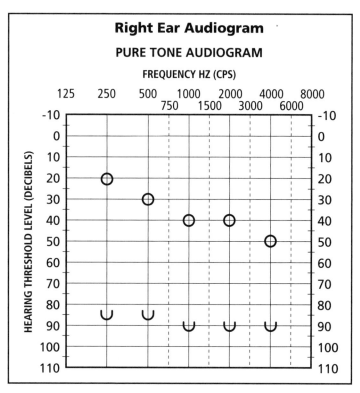

Figure 20 - Right Ear Audiogram

Loudness Growth Measurements

The audiogram in Figure 10 is characteristic of a noise induced hearing loss (noise exposure). Based upon the threshold curve and discrete UCL's, the dynamic range is wider at 500 Hz than at 3000 Hz. Therefore, the auditory area in which a hearing aid can perform effectively is wider at 500 Hz than at 3000 Hz or 4000 Hz. In fact, this generally applies to most sensorineural hearing losses as seen in Figure 9.

Figure 9 illustrates a gradual sloping hearing loss (presbycusis). The dynamic range or auditory area in the higher frequencies is narrower where the majority of speech sounds are found and more gain is required than in the lower frequencies where less gain is needed. The narrower the auditory area the more challenging it becomes to amplify comfortably in that range so as not to exceed the UCL. Advanced circuits can more effectively amplify within these narrower ranges. Loudness Growth Measurements provide a numeric system of varying intensity levels from 1 sounding

very soft to 7 sounding uncomfortably loud as seen in Figure 21.
Establishing loudness growth measurements enable clinicians
to more effectively program hearing aids so that a patient can
optimize their aided speech capability and comfort especially in
noisy environments.

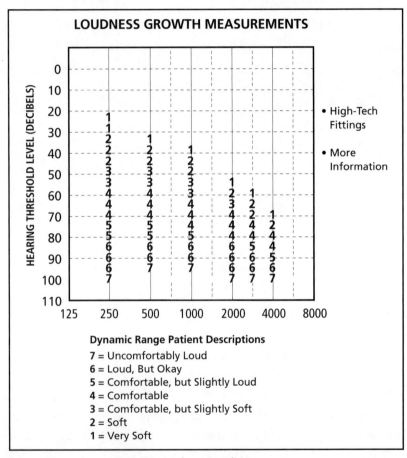

Figure 21 - Loudness Growth Measurement

Tympanometry

A comparison between air and bone conducted pure tone scores
(air/bone gap) will help determine if a hearing loss is conductive,
sensorineural, mixed or normal hearing. Tympanometry, one of
several Otoimmitance measurements, not only helps to confirm
pure tone audiometric results as it relates to the nature of a hearing
loss, it also can provide valuable information as to what may be
causing or contributing to a hearing disorder.

68

Tympanometry results are obtained by placing a metal probe covered with a soft plastic tip called the "probe tip" into the ear canal. Air pressure and low frequency tones are simultaneously introduced into the test ear. A tympanometer measures the volume of air in the ear canal, negative and positive pressure variances and also measures the compliance (movement) of the tympanic membrane. These measurements, measured in mm can help detect a number of different outer and middle ear disorders.

Generally, patients with normal hearing or sensorineural hearing loss will produce pressure variances within normal tolerances and a normal compliant tympanic membrane known as Type A tympanogram as seen in Figures 22 and 22a.

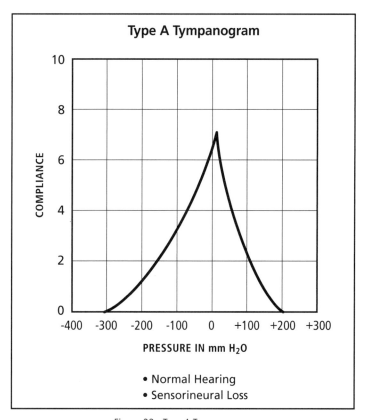

Figure 22 - Type A Tympanogram

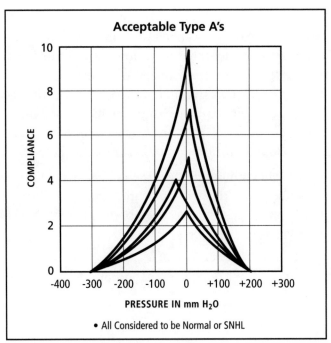

Figure 22a - Type A Tympanogram

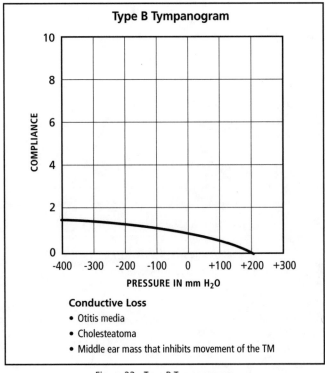

Figure 23 - Type B Tympanogram

Patients with middle ear pathology such as Otitis Media, Cholesteatoma or any condition creating a mass in the middle ear will produce abnormally negative pressure variances and a non compliant tympanic membrane known as Type B tympanogram as seen in Figure 23.

Patients developing or recovering from middle ear infection, recovering from a surgical procedure or suffering from a malfunctioning Eustachian tube will produce a Type C tympanogram as seen in Figure 24.

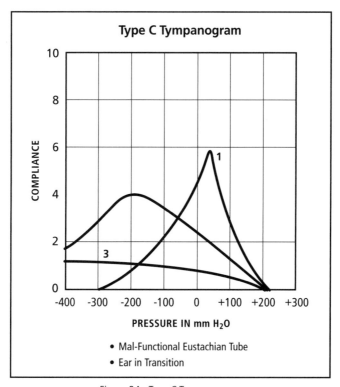

Figure 24 - Type C Tympanogram

Patients with Otosclerosis or other ossicular fixation will produce reasonably normal pressure variances and a less compliant tympanic membrane known a Type A_S (A shallow) as seen in Figure 25.

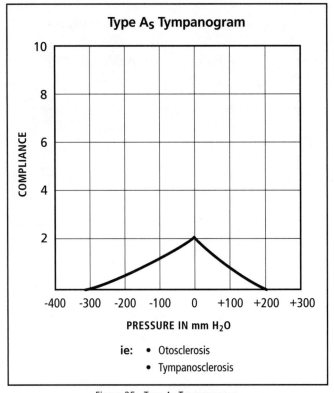

Figure 25 - Type A_S Tympanogram

An Ossicular dissarticulation, generally retracting the tympanic membrane will result in a Type A_d (A deep) tympanogram as seen in Figure 26.

Acoustic Reflex

Acoustic Reflex measurements are among the battery of Otoimmitance measurements that measure the efficacy of the Stapedius and Tensor Tympani muscles. Among the functions of these muscles is to help suspend the ossicular chain in the middle ear cavity and also protect the cochlea from dangerously loud sound by providing a damper on the system. Since the muscles in both ears respond and contract to sounds regardless of which ear

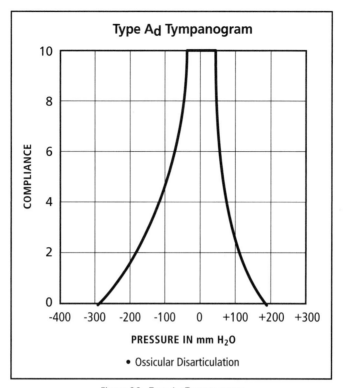

Figure 26 - Type A$_d$ Tympanogram

they are presented to, the reflexes are measured both ipsilateral (same side as signal) and contralateral (opposite side from signal). Acoustic reflex testing is important because it provides an objective assessment of the integrity of the sensory-motor pathway that crosses from one ear to the other across the lower brainstem. Abnormalities in this aural reflex can be important in determining the site of the lesion within the central auditory pathway.

Conclusion

Otoimmitance measurements assist in verifying certain audio-metric information relative to the type of disorder that may be present. It also provides information about the necessity for referral faster than any other single procedure in the customary assessment protocols.

Tuning Fork Tests

Tuning fork tests require signals to be presented via bone conduction. They provide clinicians with a quick reference relative to the nature of a hearing disorder and symmetry of a hearing loss. The result obtained from these tests will also alert clinicians as to what results they may expect from audiometric tests (Figure 27).

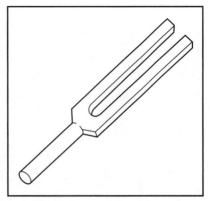

Figure 27 - 512 Hz Tuning Fork

Weber

A Weber test may reveal any one of the following three possible conditions:

1. Symmetrical hearing (same or similar hearing in both ears)
2. Ear with thresholds closest to normal hearing levels (Asymmetrical)
3. Ear with the larger conductive component

This author recommends the use of a 512 Hz tuning fork as seen in Figure 27. The tuning fork is set into vibration and the stem firmly placed to the mid-line of the patients' forehead. The patient is simply asked in which ear they hear a louder sound? If they are unable to determine which ear the sound is louder or hear the tone in the middle of their head then in all probability audiometric tests will reveal either normal hearing or a symmetrical hearing loss.

If the patient hears the tone louder on one side, one of the two following possibilities exists:

1. The tone has lateralized to the ear with hearing thresholds closest to normal hearing

Or

2. The tone has lateralized to the ear with the larger conductive component

An audiometric Weber test may also be conducted by placing the bone oscillator firmly to the patients' forehead. It is recommended that a 500 Hz pure tone signal be presented at an intensity level of 50-60 dB. Another reason for using a Weber test is to help determine which ear should be masked during bone conduction testing, in which case the ear with the larger conductive component shall be masked.

Rinne Test

A Rinne tuning fork test may provide useful information as to whether the source of a hearing disorder is conductive. Many otorhinolaryngologists routinely perform a Rinne with the assumption that their patient has a conductive hearing disorder. On the other hand, a Rinne positive would indicate either normal hearing, sensorineural hearing loss or any other pathology that may be present beyond the middle ear cavity. The result obtained from a Rinne tuning fork test is not to be interpreted as a stand alone test and must be validated by audiometric data.

As with the Weber, a 512 Hz tuning fork may be used and set into vibration. The stem of the tuning fork is held firmly to the most sensitive area of the mastoid process of the temporal bone as seen in Figure 28. When the tone is no longer heard by the patient via bone conduction the fork is held to the aperture of the test ear as seen in Figure 29. If the tone is not heard via air conduction, this indicates a conductive hearing disorder and is known as a Rinne Negative. If the tone is audible when held to the aperture of the ear canal, this indicates a Rinne Positive.

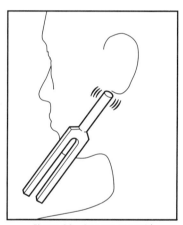

Figure 28 - Stem to Mastoid

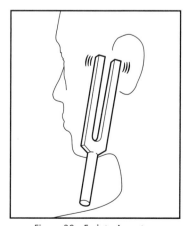

Figure 29 - Fork to Aperature

Glossary

Adipose: refers to fatty tissue such as the internal ear lobe.

Afferent: the sensory nerve fiber ascending from the end-organ toward the central nervous system.

Anterior: toward the "front".

Auricle: Latin term for "the external ear".

Basal: Latin term for "the bottom".

Basilar: referring to the lowest level or bottom layer.

Carotid: The latin name of the major artery bringing blood to the head and neck.

Caudal: Latin for "the tail" or lower.

Cerumen: The generic name for the normal exudate of the external auditory canal, it is a combination of oil and sloughed tissue.

Ceruminous: refer to the glands on the external auditory canal that produce the oil.

Chorda tympani: a branch of the nerve lying exposed in the middle ear which provides the sensation of taste to the anterior two-thirds of the tongue.

Cochlea: A "snail-shell" like structure which contains the peripheral hearing mechanisms and in which hydraulic energy is transduced into neural energy in primates. It also contains the vestibular mechanisms.

Commissure: This is a band of fibers connecting the lobes of the brain in the front or "anterior" portion.

Concha: refers to the "cavum consha" which is the depression in the external ear at the bottom of which is the opening of the external auditory meatus (canal).

Corpus callosum: refers to the thick band of fibers which connect the right and left hemispheres and is the primary site of binaural hearing.

Corti: The name of the french physician and scientist who first described the structures lying atop the basilar membrane and through which the nerve fibers pass.

Crura: Latin for "arms".

Decussation: the anatomic point at which the "cross over" of fibers in the brain stem occurs. In the auditory pathway approximately 80% of the fibers which begin on the right side "cross-over" to the left while roughly 20% remain on the same side.

Decussate: Latin for "cross-over".

Endolymph: A high sodium, low potassium electrolyte, filtrate of cerebrospinal fluid that is the fluid in which the sensory cells of both the auditory and vestibular mechanisms are located.

Epithelial: This is Latin for the outer layer of skin.

Eustachian: refers to the tube connecting the nasopharynx to the middle ear.

Fenestra ovalis: Latin for the oval window.

Fenestra rotunda: Latin for the round window.

Heschl's gyrus: This is the anatomic site on the temporal lobe in the brain at which the primary auditory area is located.

Helicotrema: This opening is located at the apex of the 2-3/4 turns of the cochlea. It is through this opening that the wave motion in the cochlea passes.

Incus: The middle of the three bones in the middle ear. It is attached between the malleus and the stapes.

Inferior: Latin for "below".

Inferior colliculus: refer to a major synapse of the auditory pathway between the lateral lemniscus and the medial geniculate bodies, which generates wave V.

Innervated: Latin for "energized" or "turned on by".

Keratin: refers to sloughed or dead skin.

Lateral: refers to "the side" or "outside" something else. Away from the middle.

Lateral lemniscus: refer to the columnar cells on the side (rising superiorly) in the brainstem which generate wave IV.

Lenticular process: refers to the lowest curved section of the incus, where it attaches to the"head" of the stapes.

Malleus: The outer most bone of the middle ear. It is attached between the tympanic membrane and the incus.

Mandible: Latin for the lower jaw.

Manubrium: this refers to the long process or "handle" of the malleus.

Meatus: Latin for canal or opening.

Medial: Latin for "toward the center".

Medial geniculate body: refers to the major synapse at the upper margin of the auditory brainstem at the level of the thalamus, between the inferior colliculus and the auditory radiation fibers which go "out" to the temporal lobes and which generate wave VI.

Medulla: refers to the anatomic structure which attaches to the pons and the junction into which the afferent branch of the VIIIth Cranial enters the brainstem.

Modiolus: refers to the central structure supporting the 2-3/4 turns of the cochlea and through which the nerve fibers pass.

Mucosa: refers to the lining of the mouth, nose, middle ear and tympanic membrane. This lining is moist and the inner layer of all of these structures.

Mucosal: referring to this layer.

Myelin: refers to the sheath covering nerve fibers.

Myelinated: indicates that the nerve is covered with this "insulating" sheath at this point.

Nasopharyngeal: refers to the area at the upper end of the pharynx and the lower margin of the nares (nose).

Nasopharynx: refers to the anatomic junction of the nares (nose) and upper throat (pharynx).

Osseous: latin for "bony".

Ossicles: refers to the three bones of the middle ear the malleus, incus, and stapes.

Otic: Latin for pertaining to the ear.

Pars flaccida: Latin for "the flaccid part" of the tympanic membrane. It refers to the upper third (which is not "stiffened" by radiation fibers) and is also called Schrapnell's Membrane.

Pars tensa: Latin for "the tense part" of the tympanic membrane. It refers to the lower two thirds which is "stiffened" by radiation fibers and is an intergral part of the impedance matching transformer action of the middle ear.

Perilymph: refers to the high potassium, low sodium electrolyte that is also a filtrate of cerebrospinal fluid and fills the membranous labyrinth of both the cochlea and vestibular mechanism.

Petrous: refers to the "most dense" bone in the body. It is the bone in which the cochlea is located.

Pinna: refers to the portion of the external ear excluding the lobule (lobe).

Pons: refers to the area between the medulla oblomgata and the brainstem, itself.

Posterior: refers to "toward the rear" or behind. It is always relative to some other structure.

Promontory: refers to the "rise" or "ridge of bone separating the oval and round windows.

Reissner's: refers to the membrane which separates the scala vestibuli and the scala media.

Resonance: refers to the frequency at which cavities vibrate most freely.

Retrocochlear: literally means "behind the cochlea" and was an early term which encompassed all lesions medial to the cochlea.

Rostral: Latin for "toward the back".

Scala media: Latin for the middle section. In the cochlea it contains the sensory cells of hearing.

Scala tympani: Latin for the portion of the membranous labyrinth from the helicotrema to the round window.

Scala vestibuli: Latin for the portion of the membranous labyrinth from the oval window membrane to the helicotrema.

Sebaceous: refers to a type of growth or cyst which contains sebum.

Shrapnell's: The physician/scientist who gave the name to the upper third of the tympanic membrane, also called the pars flaccida.

Spiral ganglia: Latin for a group of nerve cell bodies physically arranged in a spiral because of the anatomic geometry.

Spiral lamina: Latin for a "shelf of bone in a spiral orientation inside the modiolus".

Stapedius: refers to the muscle or ligament attached to it which passes from the posterior wall of the middle ear and connects to the "neck" of the stapes.

Stapes: The third and most medial bone of the ossicular chain, it is the smallest skeletal bone in the body. It is fully adult size at birth.

Stereocilia: refers to "micro hairs" which are found at the top hair cells in the cochlea. It is the bending and twisting of these hairs that cause the cells to "fire", stimulating the nerve fibers.

Stria vascularis: refers to the vascular part along the outer wall of the scala media which provides nutrients and electrical charge to the cochlea.

Superior: refers to "above" some structure.

Superior olivary complex: At the lowest levels of the brainstem the synapse is responsible for the generation of wave III.

Sylvian fissure: refers to the space (folded in upon itself) on which is located Heschl's gyrus in the temporal lobe of the brain. It is the site of the primary auditory area.

Synapse: the connection point of nerve fibers, at which axons connect to dendrites.

Tectorial: refers to the membrane (shaped like a tongue) which lies atop the stereocilia in the cochlea and which contributes to the "shearing" motion of these cells.

Tegmen tympani: refers to the thin "roof" of bone at the top of the middle ear separating it from the "floor" of the brain.

Temperomandibular: refers to the point of connection and articulation between the temporal bone and the mandible.

Tensor tympani: refers to the ligament from the other muscle of the middle ear (which arises from the area of the eustachean tube and connects on the malleus).

Tonotopicity: refers to a "one - to - one" representation.

Transduced: refers to changing energy from one kind to another.

Tragus: refers to the roughly triangular section of skin covered cartilage which is situated in front of the opening to the external auditory meatus.

Trigeminal: refers to the Vth Cranial nerve.

Umbo: refers to the process at the end of the malleus which is at the point of cone of the tympanic membrane and along it's medial surface.

Vagus: refers to the Xth Cranial nerve.

Vascular: refers to the system of blood flow.

Vascularized: refers to any organ or part having a system for the delivery of blood, nutrients or oxygen.

Vestibular: refers to the balance mechanism found in primates.